Health Education Teaching Ideas:
ELEMENTARY

Volume II

Jane Hakala, W. P. Buckner, Jr., and Karen King, *Editors*

Sponsored by the
Association for the Advancement of Health Education

an association of the
American Alliance for Health, Physical Education, Recreation and Dance

American Alliance for
Health, Physical Education,
Recreation and Dance
1900 Association Drive
Reston, Virginia 22091

ISBN 0-88314-604-5

Preface

Experts agree that the formal beginning of health instruction is essential to the development of physically, socially, emotionally, and intellectually mature students. Children of today are entitled to health information that can shape and direct the course of their lives. They are intellectually and developmentally ready to establish connections between practices and outcomes. We as educators have the responsibility to insure that young people are prepared to meet the health challenges they face in this changing society.

Subsequently, the elementary school years should be designed to develop the framework of health knowledge, reinforce positive health behaviors, and encourage skills that will facilitate healthy living. Young students need to understand that health education is an ongoing part of one's life—an area that substantially impacts each dimension of one's being. Multi-sensory learning helps students personalize and internalize health concepts and arrange them in some meaningful order for themselves. Additionally, this "hands on learning" allows students the opportunity to submerge themselves into the health curriculum.

Health education has changed dramatically over the last ten years. Health is not only a subject taught but a set of principles from which one identifies and chooses behaviors that will enhance healthy living. No longer do we rely on rote memorization, worksheets, movies, and textbooks to impart critical health information to the students. The health education learning process has evolved to actively include students in experiences that encourage the development of positive attitudes about healthful living.

We also know that attitudes about health are strongly influenced by the media, peer relationships, and societal conditions at an early age. As educators, we are actively competing with conflicting external forces to establish a "positive health mind set." One of the greatest opportunities and challenges that we face, as educators, is to successfully instill health promotion messages to the young adults of tomorrow.

There are immense opportunities for health instruction in the school setting, whether it be formal or informal. One needs to take advantage of them! The challenging part is designing learning experiences that are meaningful and relevant to the audience. Making health come alive in the classroom is not by chance but by design! This guide contains innovative learning activities and teaching ideas that will enhance classroom instruction. The materials are divided into 12 different sections which include the following topics: health content areas, health promotion, curriculum integration, and parent education.

We thank all of the health professionals who took the time to share their ideas with us.

Jane Hakala
W. P. Buckner, Jr.
Karen Douglas

Contents

HIV/AIDS PREVENTION EDUCATION

PARENT EDUCATION

PROGRAM AND INSTRUCTIONAL RESOURCES

HEALTH ATTITUDES
AND VALUES

Students in health education classes are encouraged to optimize their personal health through positive behaviors (Combs, 1983). Positive health behaviors can be defined as actions that an individual performs to enhance or maintain good health. Students who place a high value on health will practice more positive health behaviors than students who place a low value on health (Petersen-Martin, 1985). However, research has also shown that holding health in high value does not necessarily result in positive self-care behavior (Floria, 1982; Gramse, 1982). Intelligence, attitudes, decision-making skills, familial background, socioeconomic status, and the environment have the potential to influence health behavior. Personal values also have the potential to influence health behavior. Values motivate behavior because they are goal-oriented (Rokeach, 1973).

How important is it to teach children in the fifth or sixth grades about health values? Health values may seem rather remote and abstract to students unless the teacher introduces values in a creative and personal way.

The overall objective of this 50-minute lesson is first to explore the health values of the teacher, then the health values of each student by a self-reflective, written activity. The ultimate outcome of this activity is to show students the relationship between their health values and their health behavior. At the end of this activity, students will understand that they have personal ownership of their values, which ultimately motivates their behaviors.

Teaching Methods

The activity begins with a lecture demonstration at the chalkboard. The teacher introduces the activity by saying: "Today we are going to explore our health values. As you know, boys and girls, my name is Mrs. (or Mr.) _____. But today, I'm going to let you in on a secret. I'm going to tell you my first name. Does anyone know my first name?" This moment of acknowledgment is often exciting to children. For this example, the name Valerie will be used.

After making a general comment about the importance of health and wellness in her life, Valerie tapes a large letter "V" made out of construction paper onto the blackboard. She then turns to her students and says: "V stands for vigorous exercise. Daily exercise is important to me." The activity continues for several minutes until the letters spell out Valerie across the board and the identified value is written next to each letter (Table 1). Throughout the activity, Valerie describes the relationship between her personal values and her health behaviors.

†By Dr. Valerie A. Ubbes, Ph.D., C.H.E.S., Department of Physical Education, Northern Illinois University, DeKalb, IL.

Next, each student will write his/her name vertically on a piece of paper and spend 10 minutes thinking and writing health values which begin with each letter of his/her name. For example, Ann might value apples for snacks, naps, and nice friends. The teacher should move around the classroom to help students, offering suggestions to students who need assistance on their acronyms of health values. Students can also be encouraged to pair up to help one another with their last few letters. The dictionary can be used to trigger ideas when students have difficulty completing their acronyms.

In the final 10 minutes, students share their health values letter-by-letter with their partners, then volunteer "teams" are asked to share in front of the class. For example, Ed and Bill start by holding each other's acronyms for classmates to read. Ed introduces Bill and Bill introduces Ed. Using Ed and Bill as examples, the teacher reminds students about the relationship between their personal values and health behaviors. The eight steps that comprise this activity are shown in Table 2.

Materials Needed

The following materials are needed to make this activity a success: chalkboard, chalk, large block letters made out of construction paper which spells the teacher's name; masking tape; colored construction paper for each student; large felt-tipped pens for each student; and dictionaries.

Discussion

This activity encourages students to explore what they value in their lives and ultimately to reflect upon the behaviors they practice in their lives. Students can be motivated to discuss the many dimensions of health (e.g., physical, mental, emotional, social, and spiritual) in the context of their personal health values. Initially, the teacher should encourage all responses as acceptable. Because conflicts in values and behaviors may result, the teacher should be prepared to explore and discuss individual situations when they arise. For example, an overweight student named Franklin may opt to characterize the letter "F" in his name for Fat or Fatty. The teacher must be able to respond to Franklin in a sensitive way to capitalize on this teachable moment by

++

Table 1

HEALTH VALUES ACTIVITY

V IGOROUS EXERCISE

A TTITUDE

L OTS OF SLEEP

E STEEM

R ELATIONSHIPS

I NDIVIDUAL CHOICES

E ATING WELL

++

Table 2

DIRECTIONS

1. Teacher shares his/her first name with students and writes name on the chalkboard.

2. Teacher identifies a personal health value for each letter of his/her name.

3. Teacher describes the relationship between personal values and health.

4. Students write their names in a vertical column on piece of paper.

5. Students identify a personal health value for each letter of their name.

6. Students exchange papers with a partner.

7. Partners introduce one another and explain each other's health values to entire class.

8. Teacher emphasizes ownership of value systems and reinforces the relationship between value systems and health.

++

turning "borderline" health values into potentially positive behaviors. In Franklin's case, the teacher might ask him a probing question to better understand the context of his chosen value after which time a supportive response from the teacher might be: "Franklin seems willing to accept himself as being overweight, which is the first step to changing his behavior." The teacher might also need to be sensitive to cultural issues. Some Hispanic or Black persons may value "stockiness" as being healthy.

Conclusion

This activity helps students to identify and clarify some of their health values. This activity sets the foundation for future health education lessons, because students are taught that their personal values determine what behaviors they practice with regard to their health.

References

Combs, B. J. (1983). *An invitation to health* (2nd ed.). Menlo Park, CA: Benjamin Cummings.

Floria, D. L. (1982). The impact of health locus of control and health value on self-care health behavior (Doctoral dissertation, West Virginia University, 1982). *Dissertation Abstracts International, 43,* 2153-B.

Gramse, C. A. (1982). The relationship of internal-external health expectancies, value of health, health beliefs and health behavior regarding breast self-exam in women (Doctoral dissertation, New York University, 1982). *Dissertation Abstracts International, 43,* 385-B.

Petersen-Martin, J. P. (1985). *The relationship of self-concept and values to health behavior in community college students.* Masters thesis, University of Oregon.

Rokeach, M. (1973). *The nature of human values.* New York: Free Press.

UNDERSTANDING ELEMENTARY STUDENTS' PERCEPTIONS OF HEALTH THROUGH THE USE OF ARTWORK, NARRATIVE, AND CLASSROOM DISCUSSION†

This article will present the benefits of using projective techniques during elementary school health education classes to assess students' knowledge, beliefs, and attitudes about personal health. This paper is based on one part of a comprehensive community-based needs assessment completed in two rural South Carolina school districts during the spring of 1993. Research results were used to plan effective school health education instruction and health services. Middle school students illustrated or wrote about their perceptions of good and poor health and discussed their beliefs with peers. Group interviews with students permitted a more detailed understanding of students' health-related knowledge and beliefs than a quantitative paper-and-pencil questionnaire or examination.

†*By Brian F. Geiger, Ed.D., University of Alabama at Birmingham School of Education, Department of Human Studies, Birmingham, AL. This research was funded by the South Carolina Health and Human Services Finance Commission, Alternative Delivery Systems.*

The purpose of this article is to present a qualitative research method that was used as one part of a community-based case study of fifth through eighth grade students. Using student-created drawings and narratives as part of a school health class can be particularly useful to encourage participation by all students, particularly those in the younger grades who may be reluctant to speak freely in the classroom. Combining information presentation with student exercises enriches health education instruction. This teaching method can easily be used by elementary school health teachers to introduce health topics and assess students' health-related knowledge, attitudes, and beliefs before and after classroom instruction. There is only a minimal cost for instructional materials (Geiger, 1993a & 1993b).

Explanation of Teaching Idea

Students' perspectives about the meaning of good and poor health including the importance of good nutrition, physical exercise, abstention from the use of cigarettes, psychoactive drugs, and alcohol, and personal responsibility for health were revealed from their illustrations and narratives created during school health classes. The purpose of the classroom activity and ground rules were explained to students at the beginning of the class session. Two main ground rules emphasized to students were voluntary participation by individual students and respect for each student's personal beliefs and opinions including prohibition against peer criticism or censure. Ground rules were helpful to establish a nonthreatening and nonevaluative environment which encouraged disclosure (Geiger, 1993a; Stewart & Shamdasani, 1990; Beemer & Fallek, 1993). Students were provided with letter-sized unruled white paper, colored pencils, and markers. Students were asked to illustrate or write about health using a set of statements that included general and specific directions (Figure 1). For example, students were instructed to "draw or write down on your paper what the words 'good health' mean to you." Students were told that there was no right or wrong way to illustrate or write about their beliefs.

Students were encouraged to compare and contrast their personal beliefs about health by illustrating the meaning of "good health" on one side of the page and drawing the meaning of "bad health" on the opposite side of the page. Students were asked to prepare only one drawing, or write one narrative at a time. Oral directions were brief to avoid biasing participants' responses.

Following completion of the drawings or narratives, students were guided in classroom discussion about the characteristics they perceived as important to good and poor health. Students were not limited to responses to the teacher's predetermined questions, instead, questions posed by the teacher guided class discussion. Students were encouraged to describe their drawings or narratives and ask questions about personal health concerns.

The teaching idea was field tested during 7 group interviews with 96 public school students in grades 5-8; nearly all of the students were African Americans. Students were very interested in this exercise and actively participated in group discussions. Some of the students were eager to compare their completed drawings with peers. According to classroom observations and second-hand reports from teachers, students greatly enjoyed the novelty and informality of these exercises (Geiger, 1993a & 1993b).

Figure 1

SAMPLE QUESTIONS USED TO ASSESS STUDENTS' HEALTH-RELATED KNOWLEDGE AND BELIEFS

1. Draw or write down on your paper what the words good health mean to you.

2. Draw or write down on your paper what the words bad health mean to you.

3. Draw or write down on your paper what happens to somebody your age if they smoke cigarettes.

4. Draw or write down on your paper what happens to somebody your age if they drink alcohol like beer or wine.

Sample Results of the Classroom Activity for Health Education

The middle school students displayed a fundamental knowledge of good health that included eating a balanced diet and avoiding junk foods, playing sports and exercising, abstaining from tobacco, drug and alcohol use, and practicing good personal hygiene and self-care behaviors (Figures 2, 3, 4, 5, 6). Students displayed misconceptions about the physical effects of cigarettes and cocaine. Nearly all of the students emphasized a desire for social acceptance as integral to practicing positive health behaviors. Family, environmental, and mental and emotional health were significantly less often identified by students as part of what "good health" means to them.

Figure 2

SAMPLE STUDENTS' BELIEFS ABOUT THE MEANING OF GOOD HEALTH

Good health is . . .

"eating from the food groups, the meat group, the bread group, the dairy group. Bad health is eating candy bars, soda, [using] cocaine, marijuana, and crack [cocaine]. —Sixth grade female

"taking care of your body. Don't do drugs. Don't drink [alcohol]." —Sixth grade female

"bananas, little oranges, wild cherries. Bad health is liquor and cigarettes." —Sixth grade male

"She's staying in shape, now. They're exercising and happy." —Sixth grade female

---

Figure 3

ILLUSTRATION OF A FEMALE MIDDLE SCHOOL STUDENT'S PERCEPTION OF THE MEANING OF GOOD HEALTH

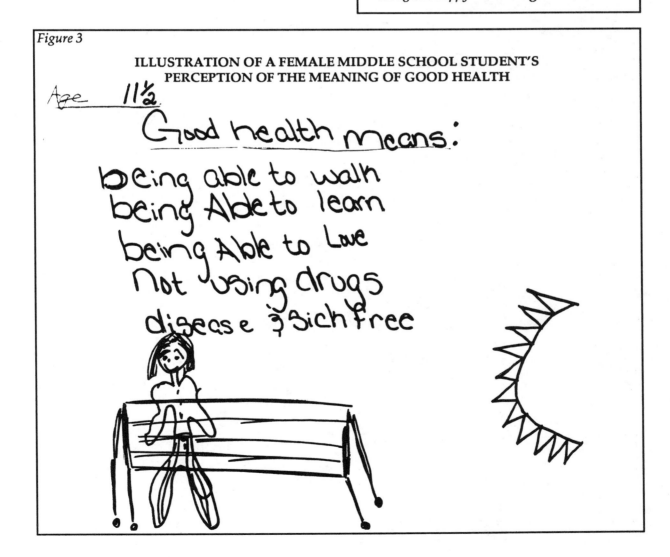

Figure 4

ILLUSTRATION OF A MALE MIDDLE SCHOOL STUDENT'S PERCEPTION OF THE MEANING OF GOOD HEALTH

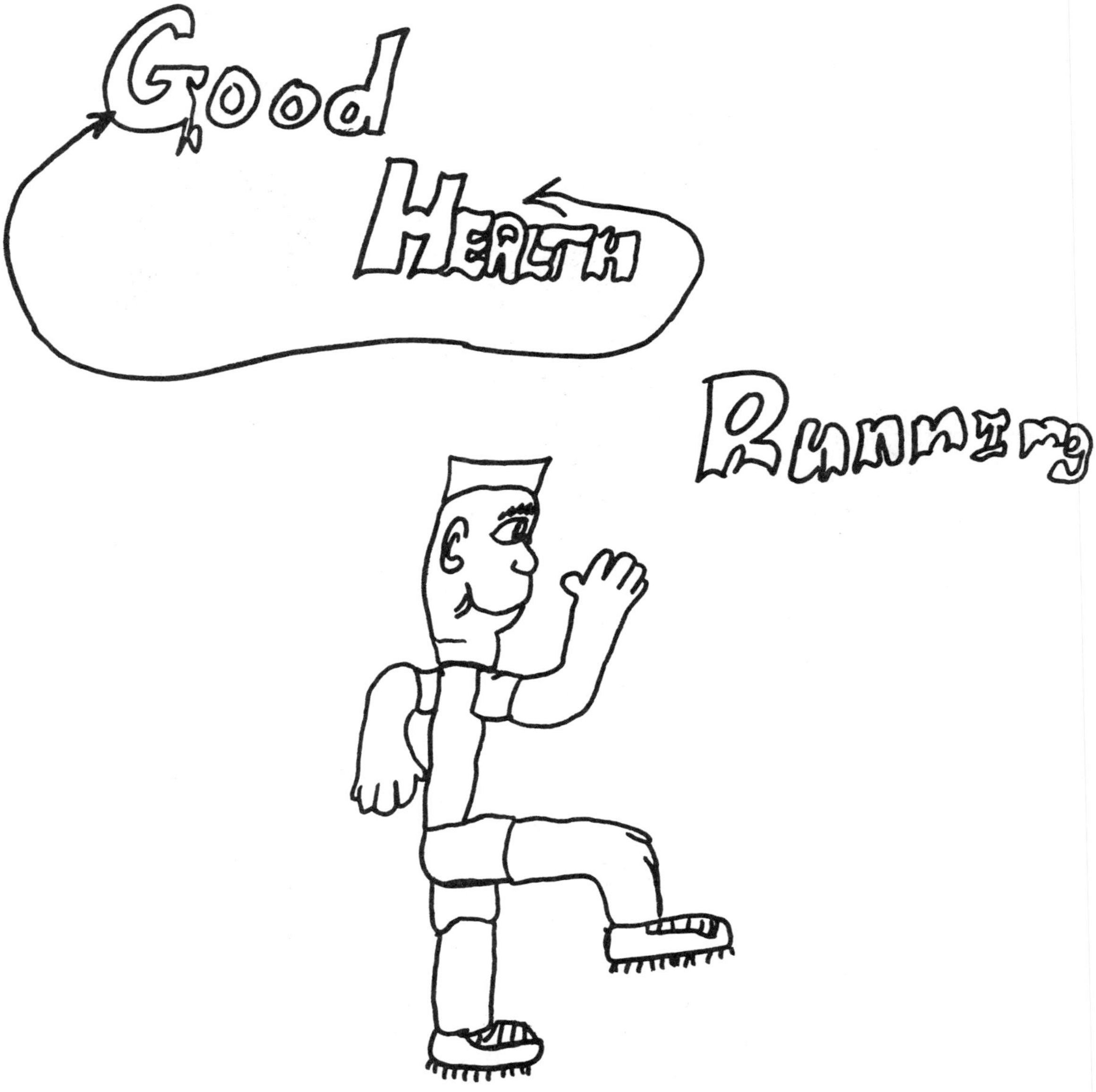

Figure 5

**ILLUSTRATION OF A FEMALE ADOLESCENT'S
PERCEPTION OF THE MEANING OF GOOD HEALTH**

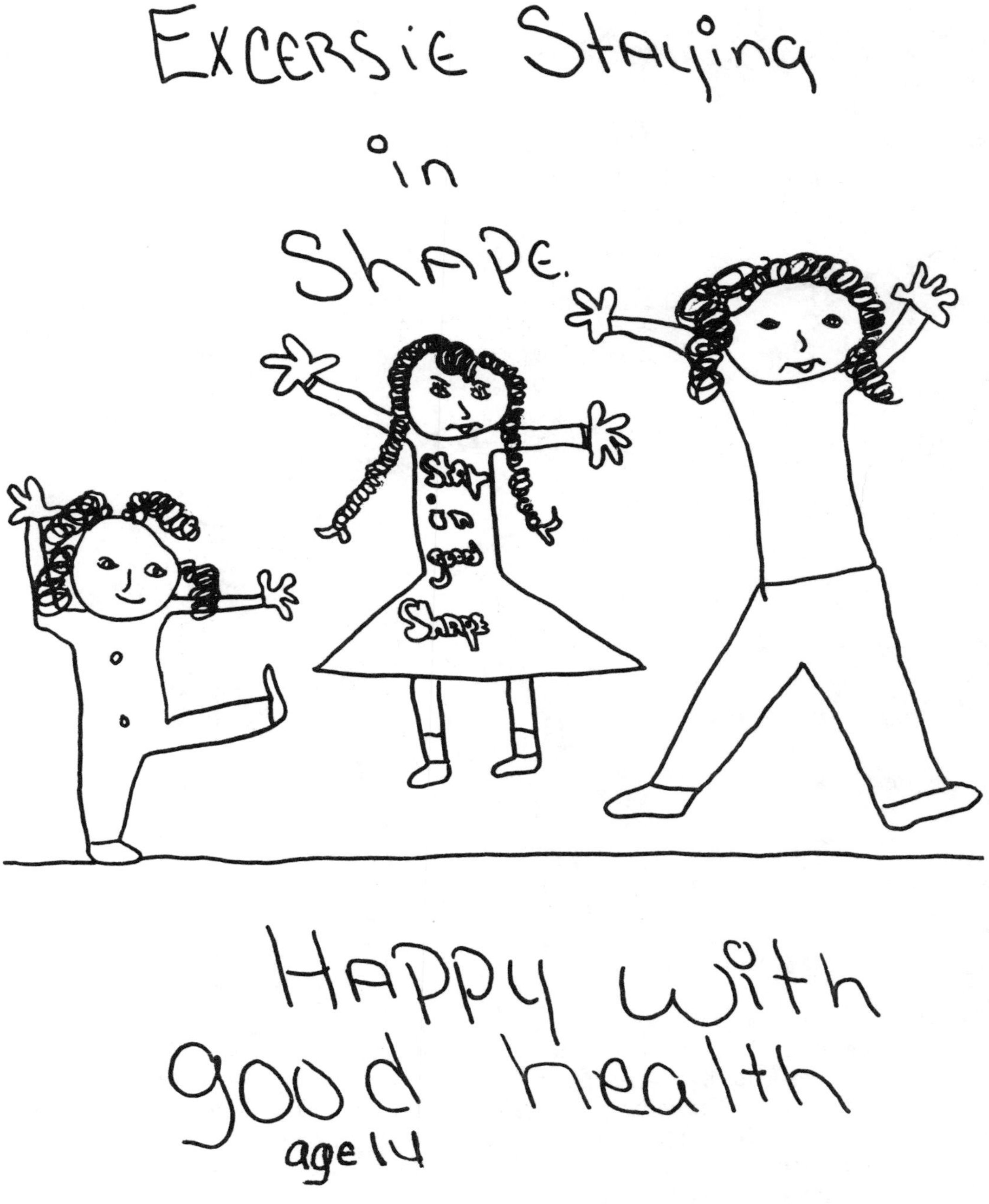

Excersie Staying in Shape.

Stay in good Shape

Happy with good health
age 14

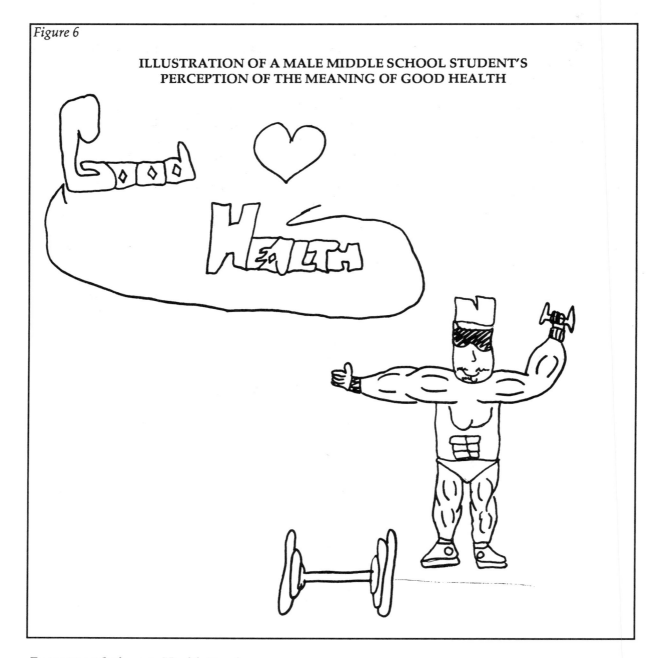

Figure 6

**ILLUSTRATION OF A MALE MIDDLE SCHOOL STUDENT'S
PERCEPTION OF THE MEANING OF GOOD HEALTH**

Recommendations to Health Teachers

Classroom teachers can further understand elementary students' unmet health education needs through projective exercises and active dialogue about health topics. This teaching idea can easily be incorporated as one exercise in an age-appropriate and comprehensive school health education curriculum. Students' drawings, narratives, and dialogue reveal their school health education needs. Students will often honestly discuss their personal health concerns and preferences for instructional content and methods for school health education if they perceive that the classroom environment is safe and the teacher is trustworthy. Comprehensive health education should occur in a sequential manner, building upon foundations taught in previous grades. The health education research literature demonstrates that such instruction can positively impact on students' health-related knowledge, attitudes, and practices (Metropolitan Life Foundation, 1988; Walberg et al., 1986; Cortese & Middleton, 1994).

References

Beemer, C. & Fallek, J. (1993, Fall). Making sexuality education relevant to young men. *Family Life Educator*, 11-15.

Cortese, P. & Middleton, K. (1994). *The comprehensive school health challenge: Promoting health through education*. Volumes I & II. Santa Cruz, CA: ETR Associates.

Geiger, B. F. (1993a). *A community case study to understand the school health education needs of adolescents for sexual risk reduction*. Doctoral dissertation, University of South Carolina, Columbia, SC.

Geiger, B. F. (1993b, November). *Understanding adolescents' perceptions of HIV and AIDS through qualitative research methods*. International Society for AIDS Education Seventh Annual Conference, Chicago, IL.

Metropolitan Life Foundation. (1988). *"Health: You've got to be taught" survey*. New York: Metropolitan Life Insurance Company, Health and Safety Education Division.

Stewart, D. W., & Shamdasani, P. N. (1990). *Basics of qualitative research: Grounded theory, procedures, and techniques*. Newbury Park, CA: SAGE Publications, Inc.

Walberg, H. J., et al. (1986). Health knowledge and attitudes change before behavior; A national evaluation of health programs finds. *ASCD Curriculum Update*, June, 4-6.

MENTAL HEALTH

BUILDING A SENSE OF COMMUNITY THROUGH FRIENDSHIP TRAINING IN THE CLASSROOM†

Teachers can help students develop a sense of community through learning situations in the classroom. Students can be taught that by accepting others and cooperating with them, they can accomplish more in their own lives while strengthening their sense of self-worth. Increasing classroom unity ultimately will lead to strengthening the community and society of which each child will become a part. Based on these concepts, the following strategies were developed to be used in the upper elementary grades (4-6).

Introduction to the Lessons

To help facilitate development of friendships within the classroom, thereby enhancing classroom unity, three activities have been developed. These activities can be utilized to help point out the uniqueness of individuals, to emphasize qualities that make a good friend, and to help nourish a sense of community and belonging.

Strategy I—We Are Not All the Same

Begin the first lesson by comparing the positive attributes of two people the students know. Possible examples would be a famous athlete and a well known political figure or a musician and the President. Talk about how these people are different, not only in looks or age, but also in lifestyle decisions, values, and personality. These differences can be listed on the board or on an overhead acetate. Contributions each makes to society should be considered and how or why these contributions are important. After using well-known subjects, bring the discussion to a more personal level by then selecting someone the students know, such as two teachers or community figures. Keeping the discussion focus on positive attributes of the individuals, talk about and list characteristics of these people that are similar and those that are different. Point out that all people have similarities and differences, and, even though they are not exactly the same, they still provide valuable input into the world of which they are a part.

Next, provide students with a worksheet (see Figure 1) and let them think of two people, such as a neighbor or family member they know. They then can list ways these people are similar and different. At the conclusion, have students write a paragraph comparing themselves with the people they have chosen.

†*By David J. Anspaugh, a professor of health sciences in the Department of HPER at Memphis State University, Memphis, TN, and Susan Hunter, an instructor in the Department of HPER at Memphis State University, Memphis. This article appeared in the Journal of Health Education, July/August 1992, Vol. 23, No. 5, pp. 304-306.*

Questions for Processing and
Closure for Strategy I

1. Are any two people you know exactly the same?

2. If people are not the same, is it possible for them to be friends?

3. If people are different, does this make one person "bad" and the other person "good"?

4. What are the qualities the people you listed in the activity have that you find particularly attractive?

Figure 1   **WORKSHEET FOR STRATEGY I**

Worksheet: Similarities and Differences

1. Think of two people you know other than friends or classmates and describe how they are alike and how they are different. Some people you can compare might be your parents, brothers, sisters, neighbors, and so on.

   Person #1 _____   Person #2 _____

   Similarities: Differences:

   1.   1.

   2.   2.

   3.   3.

   4.   4.

   5.   5.

   6.   .   6.

2. How are *you* like these people? How are you different? Write one paragraph to explain.

Strategy II—The Chain of Friendship

Review the previous strategy on how people are different, yet realize that they all can have positive qualities that make them special. Observe to the students that differences do not mean that different people cannot be friends, share, or cooperate with one another or that one is "bad" and the other is "good." Emphasize that each person can choose to view others from a positive perspective, seeing their good qualities, or negatively, focusing on what they feel are their shortcomings. When friendships develop with others, each person has someone else with whom he or she can share sorrows as well as successes. By forging strong friendships in the classroom, the spirit and unity of the class makes each student better prepared to do his or her work and face the challenges of that day. One way to strengthen the bonds of friendship in the classroom is to be able to see positive qualities in each other. Provide each student with names of three other students in the classroom and three sheets of colored construction paper (1" × 1/2" × 7").

Names should be assigned so that each student is included and will have at least three positive statements written about him or her. Have students write the names they were assigned on the construction paper. Beside each name write an important quality that person exhibits. A list of qualities can be brainstormed and written on the board before names are assigned. This will provide variety, rather than having everyone be "nice." Once finished, students take turns reading the names they were assigned and qualities observed in these people. Then staple the slips of paper together like links in a chain. All links with all names should be stapled together to make a great chain of friendship that then can be displayed in the classroom.

Strategy III—Building the Bridge of Friendship

Strategy III focuses on developing friendships with others. Walls are built between people when they see the less desirable characteristics in each other and fail to see what is good. One way to build, strengthen, and maintain friendships between people is to remind themselves of the other person's desirable qualities.

Have students count by twos and pair them with each other. Give each pair a bridge (see example) to build. Let them sign the handout, then insert words on the bridge that will strengthen their relationship. Words should emphasize positive qualities but not be "inhuman"; terms should be realistic and meaningful, such as "honest" and "easy to get along with" rather than "radical" or "awesome." Both students place words on the bridge about the other person until every plank in the bridge has been filled. When completed, bridges can be displayed in the classroom as a reminder of how to strengthen relationships.

Questions for Processing and Closure to Strategy II

1. What would happen if only three or four links were stapled together and each group of links was separate from the others?

2. Since the great chain is much longer and stronger than the pieces of chain, what are the advantages of people joining together and learning to cooperate?

3. Would you rather be part of a long chain or a short one?

4. Is it ok to have a special friend? Can we share even our special friends with others? If we do, will they still be "special"?

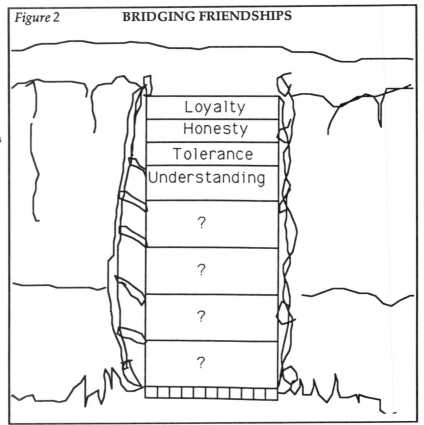

Figure 2   **BRIDGING FRIENDSHIPS**

Loyalty
Honesty
Tolerance
Understanding
?
?
?
?

Questions for Processing and Closure to Strategy III

1. What would happen if you wrote mean things about each other on the bridge? Would this make you feel good about yourselves or about each other?

2. Based on this activity, what are some of the ways you can strengthen your relationships with your friends? With your acquaintances? With other students in this classroom?

3. How are friendships built?

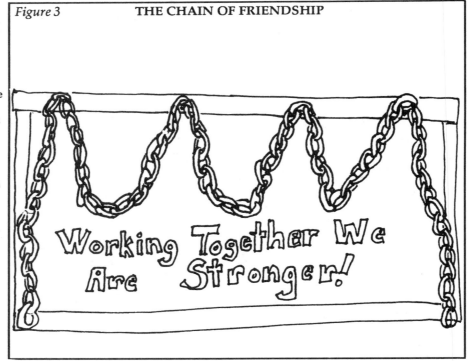

Figure 3   **THE CHAIN OF FRIENDSHIP**

Working Together We Are Stronger!

Concluding the Three Activities

To bring the three activities together and allow the student to reflect on what has been said concerning friendship and building classroom and community unity, ask students to respond to the following questions:

1. What do you consider to be characteristics of a good friend?
2. How do friendships build strength in each person? In the classroom?
3. Why is it important that people overcome their differences?

After discussing summary questions, students can list three things they have learned about one or more of the following: being a friend; characteristics friends have; why friends are important; how to form friendships; and how friendships build strength and unity. By recognizing that people are all different, by being able to accept those differences, and by looking for and emphasizing the positive in others, a solid foundation is laid for developing self esteem and recognizing each person's potential impact on the classroom, their personal environment, their community, and the nation.

THE SELF-ESTEEM AND THE SELF-CONCEPT ADVERTISEMENTS†

Grade Level: Elementary
Time Frame: One class period
Materials: Paper, paper bag, and markers

Preparation and Implementation

It has been stated that most health problems center around a poor self-concept (Curtis & Papenfuss 1980). Self-concept pertains to the mental image one has of oneself. A poor self-concept in students may be evidenced by problems related to discipline, absenteeism, substance abuse, eating disorders and suicide.

The importance of a positive self-concept in relation to the prevention of health problems is well documented. Classroom teachers can help build self-esteem by establishing classroom conditions which develop a sense of security, identity, belonging, purpose, and a sense of personal competence (Kentucky Department of Education 1989).

"Self-esteem," according to the California Task Force to Promote Self-Esteem and Personal Responsibility (1990), "is appreciating my own worth and importance and having the character to be accountable for myself and to act responsibly toward others." The commission further states, "Self-esteem is the likeliest candidate for a social vaccine, something that empowers us to live responsibly, and that inoculates us against the lives of crime, violence, substance abuse, teen pregnancy, child abuse, chronic welfare dependency, and educational failure." (1990)

According to Bean (1992), "The goal of self-esteem work is to produce learning situations in which children experience a high level of personal satisfaction at the same time as they are learning and retaining the material you're teaching them." Bean (1992) believes that self-esteem has to do with feeling satisfied while self-concept has to do with thinking about oneself. Porat (1988) indicates self-esteem grows through an inner feeling of positive self-concept and self-acceptance.

The following activities are attempts to allow elementary students to describe their feelings pertaining to self-esteem and think about positive factors associated with their self-concept. Hayes and

---

†*By Dr. Warren McNab, Professor of Health Education, College of Human Performance and Development, University of Nevada, Las Vegas, NV.*

Fors (1990) state that, "If students feel better about themselves, they may be more likely to change health-related behavior. People who feel good about themselves act more positively about their health because they feel they are worth it."

Activity 1: FOR SALE

After covering the definitions of self-esteem, self-concept, and personality, each student is assigned the task of writing a "FOR SALE" advertisement of oneself. They can choose any item and then describe characteristics that reflect their personality or self-concept.

The following are examples of advertisements students have written to describe themselves.

Advertisement One:
Kind, caring person with the personality of a rainbow
Red for strength and power
White for peacefulness and understanding
Blue for calmness and serenity
Yellow for fun and laughter
Will add vivid color to your life with goals set above the clouds and the ability to shine through
  any storm.

Advertisement Two:
I'm a fluffy, brown teddy bear, full of joy. I am just waiting for someone to pick me out of the bunch. My eyes are large with a sparkle of happiness. Happiness just waiting to be shared. My ears are open for any happy or sad tale my owner needs to express. All I ask is to be taken care of with love and affection as I will do for you.

Advertisement Three:
I consider myself a bridge—
1. Strong
2. Supportive
3. Independent
4. Giving
5. Busy
6. Stable
7. and always ending up in the middle of things.

These personality advertisements are then collected and read by the teacher to the class, keeping identities unknown. The activity should be followed by discussions on how self-concept affects the choices one makes relates to individual health. Ways to improve self-concept and the importance of a positive attitude should also be emphasized.

Activity 2: WHO ARE YOU?

A student is selected to stand and then 10 of his/her classmates ask the individual the following question, "WHO ARE YOU?" The student needs to respond with one or two words which describes their personality. Example responses might be strong, fun, happy, cool, etc. The objective is to emphasize that each person has many positive characteristics that make up their personality, and one should feel good about these unique qualities.

Activity 3: THE SELF-ESTEEM GOOD BAG

Each student decorates a large paper bag with things/drawings that represent their personality and self-concept. Then each is given blank pieces of paper, enough for each student in class, and the student must put one, anonymous positive comment about each person in class in the bag each student has made. Students are then allowed to read all the good things their classmates have said about them.

After these activities, the terms self-concept, self-esteem, and personality are reviewed emphasizing the positive feelings and thoughts one can have about themselves and others.

References

Bean, R. (1992). *The four conditions of self-esteem.* Santa Cruz, CA: ETR Associates.

California Task Force to Promote Self-Esteem and Personal and Social Responsibility. (1990). *Toward a state of self-esteem.* Sacramento, CA.

Curtis, J. D., & Papenfuss, R. L. (1980). *Health instruction: A task approach.* Minneapolis: Burgess.

Hayes, D. M., & Fors, S. W. (1990). Self-esteem and health instruction: Challenges for curriculum development. *Journal of School Health, 60*(5), 208-211.

Kentucky Department of Education: Division of Curriculum and Staff Development, Office of Instruction. (1989). *Parenting and family life skills education: A model curriculum.* Frankfort, Kentucky.

Porat, F. (1988). *Self-esteem, the key to success in work and love.* (2nd ed.) Saratoga, CA: R & E Publishers.

CREATING A TEACHABLE MOMENT IN SUICIDE PREVENTION†

Logic would dictate that in order to teach a particular lesson successfully, the health educator should know what it is that he or she is going to teach, the method to use to teach it, and how to determine if he or she has been successful. In some instances it may be important for the student or client to know these strategies as well. A well-organized teaching plan provides greater assurance that the "objectives" for the day can be met.

In addition to having a well-organized plan, health educators sometimes must prepare the student to learn. The motivation to learn is a powerful tool that, if utilized effectively, can greatly enhance learning. Educators have long touted use of the "teachable moment" as a key issue in motivating students to learn. One only has to think back to the 1986 Challenger explosion viewed by hundreds of thousands of school children. Many teachers reported that the rest of the day was spent discussing death, grief, and other issues related to the tragedy. Many teachers successfully used that "teachable moment."

While it is important for the health educator to know what he or she is going to teach, how to teach it, and how to determine if he or she is successful, there are times in which it is not advantageous for the student or client to know the primary purpose of a lesson. In addition, "teachable moments" do not occur with any regularity, and often it is difficult to depend on that to help with the teaching process. The following is an example of a powerful teaching technique that can be a lead-in on discussion about suicide, and in a way, a technique that a health educator can use to create his or her "teachable moment."

†By Mark J. Kittleson, Associate Professor in the Department of Health Education, Southern Illinois University, Carbondale, IL. Previously published in the Journal of Health Education, March/April 1994, Vol. 25, No. 2, pp. 110-111.

Starting the Activity

When you are about to start the activity, do not mention the word "suicide," or even make any suggestions that you will be discussing this topic. Make sure that your syllabus, assignments, or textbook readings do not focus on suicide.

Start off by drawing a long horizontal time line on the chalkboard. This time line will represent a person's life. At one end is birth and at the other end is death. Tell class members that they are going to create a person and his or her life. First ask class members to name the person. For this example, let's imagine that the person's name is Rachel.

After identifying Rachel as this person, ask the class to come up to the chalkboard and to mark at least two main life events on Rachel's time line. Ask students not only to identify the life event, but also to identify the age that it happened. Let students take time to identify special events. If students seem hesitant or unsure of what to put down, begin by identifying some key events, such as "getting driver's license—age 16" and "graduating from college—age 23."

It typically takes five minutes for the class to complete the timeline. Upon this line there will be many life events that Rachel has experienced. An example of a time line appears in Figure 1. (Note that Figure 1 is in a vertical format, but the activity is done best with a horizontal time line.) As you can see, students identified key events such as the day that Rachel first menstruated, her first sexual experience, her marriage, birth of children, completion of graduate school, opening of her own business, death of parents, divorce, or marriage, graduation of children from high school and college, marriage of her children, selling of business for large profit, birth of first grandchild, retirement, death of spouse, worldwide vacation, and eventually death at the age of 85.

Step Two

Now that you have described Rachel's life, go through each key issue. Ask students who wrote the key life events to describe them in more detail—for example, what did Rachel do on her first date; what was her major in college; talk about the tragedy of her third child who was born as a stillbirth and Rachel's divorce from her first husband the next year. Try to make this person as real to the students as possible. Discuss the wonders of life that include sorrow and happiness. Point out the tremendous impact that Rachel had not only on her children and spouse, but also on the many others that Rachel's life affected (friends, business associates, clients). The strategy during this step is to get the class to know Rachel as a real person, with real life problems, successes, and struggles.

Step Three

After you feel you have successfully met the requirements from step two, pick up an eraser, silently walk to the end of the time line (the death end), and start erasing both the time line, age, and life event that has taken place. Make it meticulous, slow, and deliberate. When you get to age 15 (or whatever age you decide to choose), stop erasing, take a piece of chalk, and draw a vertical line. Indicate to the class that you forgot to tell them that Rachel had an argument with her folks at the age of 15. Rachel was being grounded for staying out past her 9:00 p.m. curfew. Rachel felt the punishment was too harsh, so she killed herself. Typically, silence prevails for a few seconds at this time.

Figure 1	**TIME LINE**
Age	**Event**
85	Death
62	World cruise
60	Retirement
56	Spouse dies
53	Sells business for a large profit
51	Becomes a grandmother
46	Mother dies
44	First child graduates from high school
42	Business expands
39	Remarries
36	Father dies
33	Divorces
32	Third child born as stillbirth
30	Opening of own business
29	Second child born
28	Completes graduate school
26	First child born
24	Gets married
22	Graduates from college
19	First sexual experience
18	Graduates from high school
16	Receives driver's license
13	First date
12	Starts menstruating
10	Dog dies
5	Starts school
Birth	

Step Four

You now have an intense teachable moment. This is an excellent opportunity to discuss the effects that suicide has on the people left behind, without actually having to experience a suicide. This technique has been used with numerous groups including junior high, high school, and college. Reactions have included the following: some students were hostile and angry (they were upset that Rachel would end her life—after all, so many great things happened to her) that they actually swore at the instructor; some students expressed great sadness (several times I have seen tears well up in students' eyes); some students were in shock (in most instances the students are speechless after they find out that Rachel committed suicide); and many students simply displayed disbelief over the event ("Why would Rachel kill herself over something so stupid?"). One student even likened this activity to a modern day "It's A Wonderful Life" (a movie of the mid-1940s that showed the main character seeing the impact that his life has had on others and his community).

Although each health educator can determine how to move the lesson on, questions typically include: What was your reaction when you heard me say that Rachel killed herself? How do you think Rachel's parents, family, and friends were affected by her suicide? If you could talk to Rachel, what would you tell her?

Summary

An important part of teaching is taking advantage of teachable moments. Sometimes those teachable moments are unannounced. In some instances, you as the health educator can create your own teachable moment. When you want to discuss the impact of suicide, this activity may prepare your class to discuss the impact that suicide has among the people left behind.

GROWTH AND DEVELOPMENT

TEACHING YOUNG CHILDREN ABOUT AGING†

The U.S. population rapidly is becoming older. A child born today can expect to live to be 75 years old, 28 years longer than a child born in 1900 (American Association of Retired Persons, 1991). The older population, people 65 years or older, accounts for 31 million Americans (American Association of Retired Persons, 1991). Unfortunately, Americans often reach old age with little education or anticipatory guidance about aging and with ageist attitudes in place (McGuire, 1986).

Research has shown that ageist and ambivalent attitudes toward the elderly are evident even in preschool children (Treybig, 1974; Click & Powell, 1976; Goldman & Goldman, 1981; Burke, 1981). By the time a child is 12 to 13 years old, these ageist attitudes become difficult to change (Lorge, Tuckman, & Abrams, 1954; Bennett, 1976; Ivester & King, 1977; Burke, 1981). These ageist attitudes often become self-fulfilling prophecies in later years.

Aging education is important in helping children successfully adapt to aging. It should be intergenerational, developmentally focused, anticipatory education that promotes positive attitudes toward age and aging (McGuire, 1976). Aging education should teach children that there is potential for good health, activity, and creativity at all stages of life, and that the quality of life they will have at all ages depends largely on the decisions they make about their own lifestyle and habits (Pratt, 1987). The overall goal of aging education is to prepare youth for a long life (Pratt, 1986).

Aging education materials for children are not abundant. Two organizations that develop and catalog such materials are the Center for Understanding Aging (CUA) and Generations Together (see Figure 1). Generations Together has compiled an annotated bibliography on aging curricula for children (Wilson & Newman, 1987).

The Curriculum

In preparation for implementing aging education units with preschool children, an aging education curriculum was developed. The curriculum was juried by a panel of experts. The content of the curriculum focused on promoting healthy aging and promoting positive attitudes toward aging. The curriculum did not focus on illness, disability, or death. These topics should be dealt with separately from aging education and are not synonymous with aging. The conceptual framework shown in Figure 2 was developed for the curriculum. It actually could be implemented with aging education across the lifespan.

Figure 1

AGING EDUCATION RESOURCES

Center for Understanding Aging (CUA)
P.O. Box 246
Southington, CT 06489-0246
(203) 621-2079
Dr. Donna Couper, Executive Director
Fran Pratt, Director of Special Projects

Generations Together
University of Pittsburgh
811 William Pitt Union
Pittsburgh, PA 15260
(412) 648-7150
Dr. Sally Newman, Director
Janet Wilson, Librarian/Compiler

---

†*By Sandra L. McGuire, Associate Professor at the University of Tennessee, Knoxville, TN, and Director of Kids Are Tomorrow's Seniors (KATS Program). Previously published in the Journal of Health Education, March/April 1994, Vol. 25, No. 2, pp. 103-105.*

The curriculum incorporated early children's literature. Literature to be used in the classroom setting was screened carefully for ageism using the *Ageism in Literature* analysis form developed by Dodson & Hause (1981). A booklist of non-ageist early children's literature was developed. An updated edition of this booklist, *Non-ageist Picture Books for Young Readers: An Annotated Bibliography for Preschool to Third Grade* (McGuire, 1990), is available from the Center for Understanding Aging, as an AgeShare publication.

Figure 2   **HEALTH AND AGING CURRICULUM:**
                          CONCEPTUAL FRAMEWORK

Concept 1:   Aging is a natural and lifelong process of growing and developing.
Concept 2:   Older people and younger people are similar in many ways.
Concept 3:   Older people are valuable and contributing members of society.
Concept 4:   Old and young can enjoy each other and learn from each other.
Concept 5:   People need to plan for becoming older.
Concept 6:   People have much control over the older person they become.

Source: McGuire, S. L. (1988). *Health and Aging Curriculum—Grade Level: Preschool: Third Grade.* Eric Document reproduction service ED 291 738.

The Classroom Program

From the curriculum six teaching units were developed for implementation with preschoolers (ages four to five years). These units were implemented in a preschool program with seven locations over a tri-county area.

The units were carried out over a 3-week time period with two units being implemented each week. In keeping with the attention span for this age group, units were designed to last approximately 30-40 minutes. The children were provided with name tags for the units so that they could be referred to individually.

Unit activities were developed to be easily implemented, inexpensive, and time efficient. The units utilized discussions with the children, felt board activities, and pictures from magazines, catalogs, and newspapers. Non-ageist children's literature such as *I Know a Lady* (1984) by Charlotte Zolotow, *Miss Rumphius* (1982) by Barbara Cooney, *Song and Dance Man* (1988) by Karen Ackerman, *Good as New* (1982) by Barbara Douglass, and *The Crack-of-Dawn Walkers* (1984) by Amy Hest was used extensively throughout the units.

Unit activities focused on curriculum concepts. For example, during classroom implementation of one unit, the children were helped to understand that people aging is a natural and lifelong process. Pictures depicting people (infant through older adults) were used. The children arranged the pictures in chronological order and discussed how people grow and age, and how they were growing and aging. A children's book, *When I Get Bigger* (1983) by Mercer Mayer, was read and discussed.

It was discussed with the children that people continue to develop, learn, and do things throughout life. During this discussion the children were shown pictures of older people in a variety of activities such as jogging, swimming, dancing, going to school, working, and reading. A children's book, *Emma* (1985) by Wendy Kesselman, was read and discussed. This book depicts an older woman who begins to paint when she is 72 years old. The children talked about activities they have seen older people do, activities they thought would be fun for older people to be involved in, and activities they would like to be involved in as an older person.

In relation to planning for becoming an older person, the children talked about "lifespan" activities. Lifespan activities are activities that people can do throughout life. The children talked about present day activities that they would like to continue as older adults. Making this "lifespan" connection was fun for the children. Also, this was an opportune time for senior citizens to visit and discuss their activities.

Outcomes, Conclusions, and Recommendations

To see if attitudes about older people had changed, the children were pre- and post-tested with the Semantic Differential—Old People from the *Children's Attitudes Toward the Elderly (CATE)* (Jantz, Seefeldt, Galper, and Serock, 1976). The children's attitudes toward older people significantly improved following the teaching units.

The children's response to the units was rewarding. They eagerly participated in unit activities and frequently did not want to stop when the unit was over. They especially enjoyed the books that were read. These books provided an excellent starting point for numerous discussions about growing up and growing older. Many of the children related the characters in the stories to older people they knew.

The teachers thought that the unit materials could be easily integrated into the classroom and were pleased with the students' response. The units did not require a teacher to have an extensive background in gerontology. They required a teacher with positive attitudes about aging that could assist students in developing their own positive attitudes. Teachers were interested in obtaining the books used in the units for libraries at the preschools.

Aging education can promote more positive attitudes about aging. Children with positive attitudes toward their own and others' aging will live more fully each day and have the ability, understanding, and self-confidence to adapt to aging (McGuire, 1987). They will understand that old age can be a time of continued growth, development, and fulfillment.

References

American Association of Retired Persons. (1991). *A profile of older Americans: 1991*. Washington, DC: AARP.

Bennett, R. (1976). Can the young believe they'll get old? Attitudes of the young toward the old. A review of research. *Personnel and Guidance Journal, 55*(3), 136-139.

Burke, J. L. (1981). Young children's attitudes and perceptions of older adults. *International Journal of Aging and Human Development, 14*(3), 205-221.

Click, E., & Powell, J. (1976). *Preschool children's perceptions of the aged*. ERIC Document Reproduction Service ED 149 849.

Dodson, A. E., & Hause, J. B. (1981). *Ageism in literature: An analysis kit for teachers and librarians*. Acton, MA: Teaching and Learning About Aging Project. Acton-Boxborough Regional Schools. (Now available through the Center for Understanding Aging).

Goldman, R. J., & Goldman, J. D. G. (1981). How children view old age and aging: A developmental study of aging in four countries. *Australian Journal of Psychiatry, 33*(3), 405-408.

Ivester, C., & King, K. (1977). Attitudes of adolescents toward the aged. *Gerontology, 17*(1), 85-89.

Jantz, R. K., Seefeldt, C., Galper, A., & Serock, K. (1976). *The CATE: Children's Attitudes Toward the Elderly. Test manual*. College Park, MD: University of Maryland. ERIC Document ED 181 081.

Lorge, I., Tuckman, J., & Abrams, A. R. (1954). Attitudes of junior and senior high school students toward aging. *Annual Report of the New York Joint Legislative Committee on the Problems of Aging*, 59-63.

McGuire, S. L. (1986). Promoting positive attitudes toward aging among children. *Journal of School Health, 56*(8), 322-324.

McGuire, S. L. (1987). Aging education in schools. *Journal of School Health, 57*(5), 174-176.

McGuire, S. L. (1988). *Health and aging curriculum. Grade level: Preschool-third grade*. (ERIC Document Reproduction Service ED 291-738).

McGuire, S. L. (1990). *Non-ageist picture books for young readers: Annotated bibliography for preschool-third grade*. Southington, CT: Center for Understanding Aging (Age Share Publication).

Pratt, F. (1986). Aging education aim: Prepare youth for long life. *Perspective on Aging, 15*(2), 4-5.

Pratt, F. (1987). Teaching today's kids—Tomorrow's elders. In Harold Cox (Ed.), *Aging* (5th ed.), pp. 93-99. Guilford, CT: Dushkin Publishing.

Treybig, D. L. (1974). Language, children and attitudes toward the aged: A longitudinal study. *Gerontologist, 14*(5), p. 75. (Abstract of a paper presented at the meeting of the Gerontological Society, Portland, OR).

Wilson, J., & Newman, S. (1987). *An overview of curricula on aging and intergenerational programs for preschool to grade 12: An annotated bibliography*. Pittsburgh, PA: Generations Together.

TEACHING THE DEVELOPMENTAL PROCESS TO ELEMENTARY CHILDREN†

Family life education is probably the most controversial subject for which a teacher is asked to provide instruction. Effective family life education seeks to develop an understanding and appreciation of self and members of the opposite sex, and to promote the responsibilities of functional family living. A family life program should begin early in the child's school experience and be more fully developed each year. This type of program at the elementary level can be justified based on the natural concern that children have for the developmental process at that age.

The school classroom setting serves as a place where reliable and accurate family life information can be presented in a non-threatening, open atmosphere. Teachers must be very sensitive to their own biases and personal qualifications before undertaking sex education in order for objective material to be presented. Bruess and Greenberg (1981) recommend that the following criteria serve as qualifications for sex educators:

1. The teacher must have come to terms with his or her own sexuality, and have admitted not only to its existence but to its full status in the dynamics of his or her total personality functioning;

2. The teacher needs to know the appropriate factual material associated with the subject matter that he or she is to teach;

3. The teacher of sex education needs to be able to use the language of sex easily and naturally, especially in the presence of the young;

4. He or she needs to be familiar with the sequence of psychosexual development events throughout life; and,

5. The teacher needs an acute awareness of the enormous social changes that are in progress and of their implications for changes in our patterns of sexual attitudes, practices, laws, and institutions. These qualities will help to minimize embarrassment when teaching sex-related materials.

One area many teachers are hesitant to discuss is that of the developmental process. This may represent a serious concern to the teacher, particularly in the elementary school. Yet this is a natural area of interest and concern to students, especially those in the upper elementary grades. To aid the teacher in acquainting students with the developmental process, the writers have modified an activity originally developed by Planned Parenthood of Memphis. This activity may be taught either in mixed groups or by separating the sexes. It is the feeling of the writers that the activity be taught in co-educational situations whenever possible; however, the activity may be adapted easily to individual teachers' situations.

The 'Body Timetable' can be used to help children understand what is happening to their bodies. It is suggested that the teacher introduce the subject by discussing how everyone follows schedules and how, at certain times, various activities take place. For example, throughout the school day's schedule, reading, math, or physical education is taught at a prescribed time. Relate to the class that the body also has a timetable or schedule for maturation events to occur. The writers suggest that the teacher then proceed with a discussion regarding the fact that girls' timetables are slightly ahead of those of boys.

The teacher should introduce the 'Body Timetable' to the class and ask them to place a number in the square to show what order the body events occur. After the students have completed the timetables, the teacher can more fully explain each event and the correct order in which the events usually occur. Discussion and questions should be encouraged. One way of stimulating discussion would be to give each student an index card and allow each child to write questions anonymously on the cards to be addressed by the teacher.

†By David J. Anspaugh, professor in the Division of Health Science and Safety Education, Memphis State University, Memphis, TN, and Gene Ezell, associate and distinguished professor, Health Education, University of Tennessee at Chattanooga, Chattanooga, TN. Previously published in Health Education, March/April 1984, 15(2), 44-46.

This is an excellent introductory activity to help both the group and the teacher feel at ease. It also provides much needed information for fourth through sixth grade children. The activity is a good springboard for further discussion to help students become aware of the physical signs of reaching reproductive maturity.

The onset of puberty varies widely (boys from age 10 to 14, and girls from age 8 to 12). It may be necessary for the teacher to discuss the more subtle changes and how the beginning stages often go unnoticed. For the student, the activity and discussion provides assurance that all the changes do not take place all at once, but rather occur over a period of time. The correct order of change is provided on the 'Body Timetables' shown in Figures 1 and 2.

This activity was adapted from a larger curriculum developed by Planned Parenthood of Memphis under a grant from the U.S. Department of Health and Human Services. The curriculum contains over 40 activities and includes a series of films designed to promote discussion and decision-making. Further information can be obtained by writing Ms. Barbara Feibelman, Educational Coordinator, Memphis Planned Parenthood, 1407 Union Avenue, Memphis, Tennessee, 38152.

Reference: Bruess, C. E., & Greenberg, J. S. *Sex Education: Theory and Practice*. Belmont, CA: Wadsworth Publishing Company, 1981, p. 31.

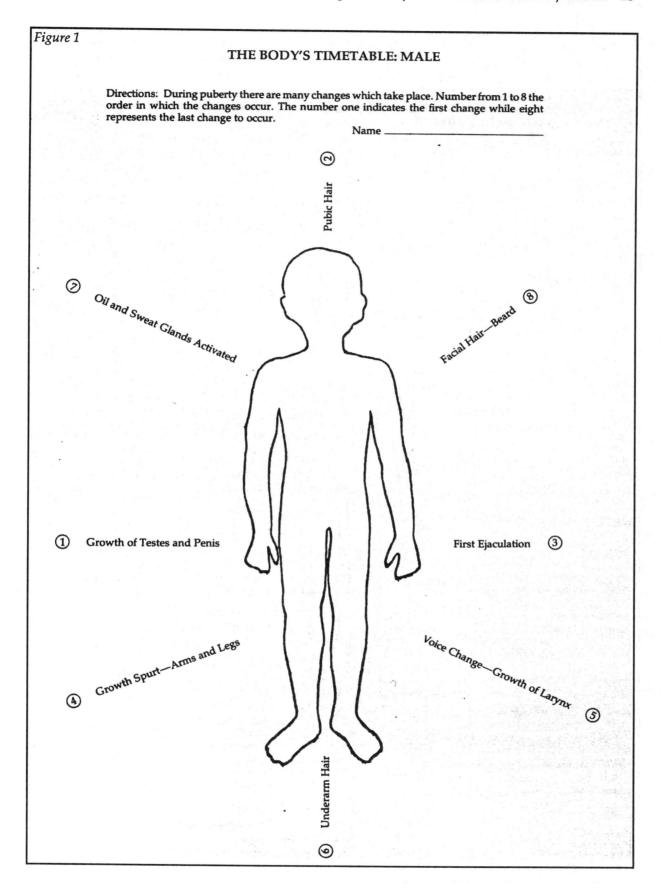

Figure 1

THE BODY'S TIMETABLE: MALE

Directions: During puberty there are many changes which take place. Number from 1 to 8 the order in which the changes occur. The number one indicates the first change while eight represents the last change to occur.

Name _____

② Pubic Hair

⑦ Oil and Sweat Glands Activated

⑧ Facial Hair—Beard

① Growth of Testes and Penis

③ First Ejaculation

④ Growth Spurt—Arms and Legs

⑤ Voice Change—Growth of Larynx

⑥ Underarm Hair

Figure 2

THE BODY'S TIMETABLE: FEMALE

Directions: During puberty there are many changes which take place. Number 1 to 8 the order in which the changes occur. The number one indicates the first change while eight represents the last change to occur.

Name _____

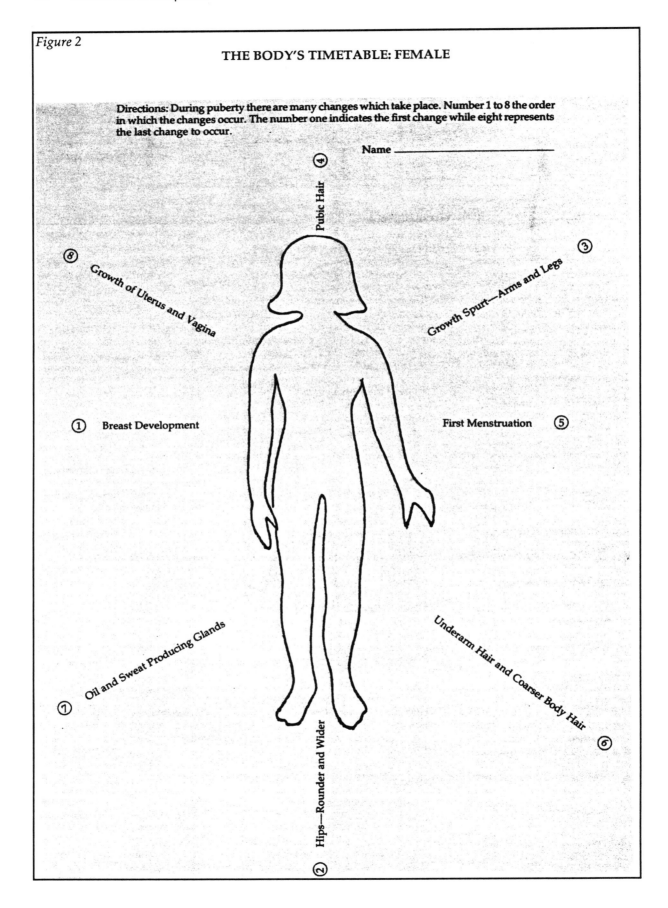

④ Pubic Hair

⑧ Growth of Uterus and Vagina

③ Growth Spurt—Arms and Legs

① Breast Development

⑤ First Menstruation

⑦ Oil and Sweat Producing Glands

⑥ Underarm Hair and Coarser Body Hair

② Hips—Rounder and Wider

UNDERSTANDING THE DIFFICULTIES OF THE DISABLED: A CLASS ACTIVITY FOR ELEMENTARY STUDENTS†

Introduction

At one time or another most people will experience some type of disability—a broken arm, hearing loss, visual impairment. Whether temporarily disabled or permanently handicapped or "differently abled," the total population coping with disability is quite large and increasing as society ages (Ebersole & Hess, 1990). This growing segment has made us more aware of the difficulties involved in daily life for those who do not have full use of their limbs or senses.

Children can be made aware of these limitations through educational activities that allow them to personally experience some aspects of the lifestyles of the disabled. All too often our educational experiences are limited to the cognitive domain, where we read or hear about situations or people. Activities like the following, which involve the affective domain, allow us to learn through personal experiences. It is a simple activity that can be easily implemented and is adaptable for many age groups, especially third grade and up.

The Setup

This activity can take place in any classroom that can be rearranged to allow for four stations. The best way to set up the room is to put the stations in the corners, with the wheelchair activity conducted in the center of the classroom. Materials required for this activity include a television; blindfolds (approximately six); six pairs of household rubber gloves or any type of gloves other than surgical gloves; a box of cotton balls; a 10-12' piece of any type of rope; 2-3 wheelchairs; and a variety of objects with different types of surfaces and shapes, such as sandpaper, an orange, paper clips and a small box.

The Process

Divide the class into four groups, with each group starting at a different station and rotating through the four stations in order. In order to facilitate groupings and maximize class time, the teacher may give each student a piece of paper bearing a number as they enter the classroom. This number will be their group number, as well as the number of their first station. Groups can then precede in numerical order.

Each station's activity will require about eight minutes, with time variances depending on the number of students and groups. The entire activity, including discussion, can be accomplished in a 50-minute class period.

Station 1—Hearing Deprivation. Have each student put cotton balls in their ears. Turn the television on without the sound.

Station 2—Sight Deprivation. Blindfold each student except one, who will become the leader. Each of the blindfolded students will hold onto a section of the rope, with the leader at the beginning. The leader will walk around the room, leading the blindfolded students.

Station 3—Tactile Deprivation. Each student dons a pair of gloves and touches the sandpaper and orange, experiencing different sensations. To test dexterity they can pick up the paper clips and attempt to put them into the box.

Station 4—Mobility Deprivation. A student sits in a wheelchair, acting the part of a paraplegic, paralyzed from the waist down. The student then attempts to negotiate a row of chairs or desks, with the row snaking, curving and eventually narrowing.

---

†By Vivien C. Carver, Ed.D., Associate Professor Community Health, The University of Southern Mississippi, Hattiesburg, MS.

Discussion

After each group has completed all four stations, a classwide discussion is held. Questions are asked about the activities at each station. Appropriate questions include: How did you feel at each station? What station presented the most difficulty? the least? Which disability do you think would be the hardest to live with? Why? Which disability would be the easiest to live with? Why?

Discussion should also center around these questions: When you see a disabled person, how should you interact with them? Has this exercise changed your perception of the disabled? How?

Conclusion

While this activity provides a great deal of enthusiasm and physical participation, it also allows students to understand the difficulties experienced by the disabled. The tremendous amount of discussion generated causes students to examine their beliefs and attitudes about handicapped individuals. Hopefully, the students will develop empathy for the disabled and an appreciation for their own healthy bodies.

Reference

Ebersole, P., & Hess, P. (1990). *Toward healthy aging: Human needs and nursing response.* St. Louis, MO: C. V. Mosby Publishing Company.

WHEN A CHILD IS BORN†

The birth of a child should be a celebrated event. Social issues such as abortion, overpopulation, and teenage pregnancy divert attention from the positive aspects of childbirth. Health educators can play a constructive role in promoting a comfortable attitude about pregnancy and childbirth, and dispel some of the misgivings, varied perceptions, and fears that children develop.

One of the most intriguing ways to experience childbirth vicariously in the classroom is to simulate the birth of a child. This lesson focuses on five major objectives: (1) to observe the birth of a child, (2) to develop a knowledge of the stages in the birth of a child, (3) to participate in the celebration of the birth of a child, (4) to present behaviors that represent a healthy prenatal environment, and (5) to engage pupils in activities related to raising a baby healthfully and lovingly.

This activity is suitable for elementary grade levels; however, the scope and detail of the content will vary. Suggested prerequisite or follow-up activities are listed.

Materials

Materials needed for this activity include a turtleneck sweater, two cabbage patch dolls, a hospital gown, stethoscope, doctors' and nurses' green gowns, face masks, hair caps, and rubber gloves. Additional detail can be included such as a water filled balloon, and red socks stuffed with other socks.

Procedure

The children have been alerted of the mother's due date. As the date approaches, anticipation and preparation increases. Energy and excitement builds. Parents are informed about this unit and invited

†*By Andy Anderson, instructor of physical and health education, University of Western Ontario, London, Ontario.*

to observe and share in class activities and discussions. A pregnant mother might volunteer to come to class to let the children hear about how it feels to have a baby inside someone Feeling the baby kicking is an exciting sensation. The children also will be learning about stages of development of the baby in the womb, what to expect in terms of needs of the mother, and how the rest of the family can help.

When the mother goes into labor, the birthing session begins. Perhaps just before recess, tell the children the mother has gone into labor a few hours ago, and when they return to class the mother will be brought in by ambulance for this event.

This activity basically is role playing or simulation. A student volunteers to be the mother. Put the two dolls inside the sweater, along with the red socks (placenta) and the water balloon (amniotic fluid). Turn the sweater upside down and tie it to the child. Cover this with a hospital smock, then don your own hospital greens and face mask. Another child may wish to be the father who has chosen to be present. Soft relaxing music may be played to show the children that the environment of a birthing room is a warm, friendly place. Ultimately, the detail presented during the birthing is determined by the teacher.

Eventually the babies emerge. You need to manipulate the dolls physically so that birth is head first, but breach birth can occur. Dolls are brought out by hand and given to the mother. Surgical cord can be attached to represent the umbilical cord and can be cut to explain the belly button. The excitement shared in this experience is amazing. Students all want to hold the baby, wrap it up, and put it in the cradle they have meticulously prepared. Sometimes, as a reward, a student can take home the class baby for a night.

Perceptions about pregnancy and how babies are born serves as a good lead-up to the event. Anatomical outlines provide appropriate terminology and vocabulary. Math classes can do some catalogue purchasing of baby essentials and calculate yearly costs associated with child care. Language arts classes can prepare congratulatory cards, birth announcements, and organize a birthday party. In primary classes the materials can be left at a center for children to use later. Discussions about the stages of fetal growth can help to solve mysteries about pregnancy. How humans are born and cared for can be compared to how other mammals bear, nurture, and care for their young. Students also may study and keep track of changes a baby goes through the first year. For example, weight, length, ability to track objects visually, the ability to grasp, foods consumed, and so on relate well to many other subject skills. These results may be compared to ways in which other animals mature and why the human process is different.

Extension activities include care and feeding of a baby. Health nurse and parent presentations serve to demonstrate community concern and respect for babies. Members of the religious community should be invited to share their traditional practices in the celebration and ceremony of children in the church, e.g., baptism. Discussions regarding the rights of children promote integrity and enhance self-esteem. A visit to the hospital and maternity unit will inspire discussions and consolidate concepts.

Older children can benefit from babysitting courses, infant nutrition, and exercise instruction. Play activities, toy design, and selection ideas can be distributed through newsletters to parents. Often classrooms or whole schools will adopt a child from a third world nation. Funds raised are sent to provide clothing, food, and educational materials. Appreciation of our global responsibility and concern for children is an important aspect of citizenry.

This activity is a rich opportunity to show males that the responsibility of caring for the baby can be shared by both mother and father.

I have found that this unit is a time to share warm feelings about family members and events surrounding the birth of younger brothers and sisters, cousins, and even neighbors. Also, class discussions abut family ancestry integrate well with social studies activities. This unit can help children who are in blended families become a little more relaxed about their situation and realize how much they are loved despite their circumstances. Although the birth is the "main event," the children soon realize that it is part of a much larger concept.

A note to parents before this event may prevent embarrassing questions. Also parents may alert you to special situations such as adoption that may influence presentation of your message.

ANATOMY
AND PHYSIOLOGY

HUMAN ANATOMY AND PHYSIOLOGY: UNDERSTANDING THE GASTROINTESTINAL SYSTEM[†]

Grade Level: 2-4

Time Frame: 35 minutes

Materials: Rolls of butcher paper (ideally in colors white, red, yellow, and green), scissors, colored marking pens, construction paper, and masking tape

Background Information

Even before the publication of the SHES study in 1967, the understanding of the human body as a vital component of health education was well established (Green, 1990). As a part of this on-going health education emphasis in the school setting, the gastrointestinal system (aka Digestive System) is one of ten basic body systems that is taught in the elementary grades (Bender & Sorochan, 1989).

This activity is designed to act as either an introductory or summary activity. Depending upon the readiness of the learners, teaching about this system can be limited to the basic parts (mouth, esophagus, stomach, small intestine and large intestine) or expanded to include the "companion" organs (gall bladder, pancreas, and liver). The materials can be prepared by either the classroom teacher, or can be a class project leading up to the strategy delineated below. The activity can be adapted easily for students with special needs whether physical or mental in nature. The major objective of the activity is to allow the students to obtain an understanding of the gastrointestinal system through a digestion simulation.

Preparation

Select the number of organs involved in your model. (In this illustration, four are used.) Assign the parts to four groups of students. The students with the mouth cut white butcher paper long enough and wide enough to cover the door to the classroom. The paper should be slit in the middle to allow for student groups of four or five to pass through without ripping the paper. The design on the sheet should be an open mouth showing teeth, gums, and tongue. Written on the sheets are two or three major functions of the mouth A second group prepares a long (red) esophagus that can be placed upon the floor and wide enough for individual students to walk upon. The same "function rule" applies with the esophagus as it did with the mouth. A third group of students prepares a stomach model (e.g., on green paper) large enough for 5 to 10 students to stand upon at one time.

[†]*By Dr. Charles Regin, Assistant Professor of Health Education, School of HPER, University of Nevada, Las Vegas, NV.*

Again, the functions of the stomach are written upon the sheets. The final student group creates a large intestine/small intestine model (e.g., on yellow paper). The model should be large enough to allow students to walk upon the intestinal system from start to finish. The functions of both systems are written in appropriate areas. If more organs are used, they should be placed appropriately on the outside perimeter with functions listed. It is then decided by the students or teacher which foods are going to be "digested." Once determined, the major nutrient components of that food item must be identified (e.g., a slice of enriched bread = protein, carbohydrates, potassium, and niacin). These nutrients are written on sheets of paper which can be taped to student clothes. Before the start of the lesson, the four model components are attached to each other leading from the classroom door and concluding in the middle of the classroom floor.

Implementation

Four or five students are assigned to be a food item. The single sheets of nutrient components of the food are taped to each student. Each food item group then bunches close together outside the classroom door. To begin the process, the students read aloud the function information. The students then proceed through the mouth and are "broken up" into individual parts and proceed single file into the stomach. Depending upon the size of the stomach, one or more food items can be "chewed and swallowed." (*Teacher note:* Various additional informational items can be presented by the teacher as this activity progresses.) In the stomach, the digestive process continues as students remove the sheets from their clothing that are affected by stomach acids. Each student then passes into the small intestine where the food item sheets are further digested or "absorbed" (i.e., the nutrient sheets are given to students who are standing around the model who represent cells or the blood stream). If other digestive organs are used, then sheets representing their digestive hormones (e.g., insulin, bile, etc.) should be given to the "pieces" of food for appropriate response. The students then move into the large intestine, any final nutrients (e.g., water) are absorbed, and the remains "move out of" the model.

Variations

Combinations with other body systems (e.g., circulatory) can be accomplished to trace the route of the nutrients. Each system can have its own model created and students can role play the active components of each specific system. The activity can be easily integrated into other academic areas (e.g., science). In addition, body systems are basic and can, depending upon the readiness of the students, be taught with either a great deal of information or using limited detail.

References

Bender, S. J., & Sorochan, W. D. (1989). *Teaching elementary health science.* Boston: Jones and Bartlett. Green, L. W. (1990). *Community health.* (6th edition). St. Louis: Times Mirror.

"DIGESTING" HEALTH INFORMATION†

Ideally, health educators are in a state of never-ending search for better methods. Sharing is bound to be the best contributor to this search.

In sharing, the author has found this play to be a highly motivating approach to the teaching of the digestive system. "What Happened to the Apple" is geared toward upper elementary aged students, but works quite well with "low achieving" junior high school students. Audience participation allows all class members to become involved and interested.

After the narrator closes the play, students may want to try different roles. The play takes no more than five minutes to perform and can easily be repeated. Hopefully, students will memorize the apple's path with enthusiasm.

What Happened to the Apple?

Characters: Apple, Stomach, Small Intestine, Large Intestine, Mouth and Teeth, and the entire audience.

Apple: That girl just picked me up. Oh No!

Mouth and Teeth: Let's grind this apple into small pieces so the stomach won't have to do it. Teeth, when you're finished, have the tongue move the smaller pieces to the throat. Mouth, you turn on your hoses and wet this food down with saliva so that the throat won't complain when it swallows.

Apple: It sure is dark in here! Where am I anyway?

Audience: You, apple, are in the stomach! and You look more like applesauce after what the mouth and teeth did to you.

Apple: But how did I get here?

Audience: You came down the esophagus!

Stomach: Oops! Looks like my rest is over. I've got to get busy and digest more food. It sure is rough work breaking up carbohydrates and protein. But, at least there is no fat coming in this time. I hate breaking up fat!

Audience: Hey, stomach. Do you like your job?

Stomach: Most of the time my boss treats me pretty well, but every now and then he delivers the wrong kind of food and I go on strike!

Apple: Whoo! Where am I going now? What's happening to me?

Audience: Don't you know apple? Your time in the stomach is up now; you have to go to the small intestine.

Small Intestine: I can't wait to absorb you into my blood, apple!

Apple: But what will happen to me when I'm in your blood?

Small Intestine: Your carbohydrates will be burned for energy and your protein can be used for growth and repair of the body.

Audience: Hey small intestine! How are you going to absorb the apple?

Small Intestine: Well, I must admit, it won't be an easy task. I'll have to have help from my friends, Liver and Pancreas.

Apple: There's not much of me left! But I'm still here. The small intestine didn't use all of me. I still have my roughage and some of my water.

Audience: Here comes the large intestine.

Large Intestine: I'm gonna be glad to get that apple in me—I like roughage. I'll soak up that leftover water as well.

Narrator: The large intestine did soak up the apple's leftover water. Then the large intestine compacted and eliminated the roughage from the body. The body was grateful to the apple for providing so many good nutrients.

---

†*By Richard A. Crosby, Department of Health Education, Central Michigan University, Mt. Pleasant, MI. The article was previously published in Health Education, April/May 1986, 17(2), 52.*

TEACHING CHILDREN TO PROTECT AND CONSERVE THEIR HEARING†

As long as environmental noise—from motorcycles, personal headphone stereos, airplanes, and shop tools, among other sources—threatens the hearing health of children, adolescents, and adults, elementary school teachers will need to teach children about hearing health and conservation. And whenever teaching is the topic, two questions always will be raised: (1) what should be taught? and (2) how should it be taught? This article suggests answers to these questions of hearing health curriculum and method.

Curriculum

There is a lot of agreement, at least among authors of health textbooks, about what should constitute the elementary school hearing health curriculum. In general, this curriculum can be divided into five categories of information:
> (1) the physical process of hearing
> (2) the nature of sound
> (3) what noise is and why it is a concern
> (4) signs and causes of hearing problems
> (5) how to protect one's hearing.

Within each of these five areas of the curriculum is a set of concepts which define the content, that is, what is usually taught. Examples of concepts in each of these five areas are presented in the diagram below:

I. *Hearing Process . . .*
   Ear has three parts (diagram of ear)
   brain interprets sounds from ears

II. *Nature of Sound . . .*
   is air moving or vibrating
   is wave motion
   varies in loudness and pitch
   loudness is measured in decibels
   insulating materials reduce loudness

III. *Noise . . .*
   can damage health
   can disturb sleep, cause stress, headaches
   is considered pollution if excessive
   is caused by traffic, appliances
   can be fought by laws
   can be reduced at home

IV. *Hearing Problem . . .*
   signs include pains in ears, buzzing,
      difficulty in hearing
   causes include colds, infections, germs,
      too much ear wax
   causes include excessive noise

V. *Protect Hearing by . . .*
   turning down TV and radio
   not sticking things in ears
   washing ears
   wearing hearing protection
   hearing check-ups (doctors and nurses
      look in ears, use audiometer and
      otoscope)

While the concepts listed above can be thought of as a starting point or basic curriculum for teaching hearing health, there are many more concepts that could also be included in a complete hearing health curriculum. Listed below are some additional concepts to consider:

---

†By Alan M. Frager, Associate Professor in the Department of Teacher Education, Miami University, Oxford, Ohio. The article was previously published in Journal of Health Education, July/August 1992, 23(5), 310-311.

(1) Pain does not always accompany hearing loss.
(2) Mild hearing losses can create frustrating communication situations.
(3) A person might not know if he or she has a noise-caused hearing problem.
(4) There are many different kinds of hearing loss.
(5) An audiologist is a person who works at identifying and preventing hearing problems.
(6) Audiograms tell a lot about a person's hearing health, but not everything about it.
(7) Hearing protection is worn by workers in many professions, including: construction, airline work, landscaping, and the military.
(8) Hearing impairment ranges from mild loss of hearing to total deafness.
(9) Hearing aids gather sound, electrically intensify it, and channel it to the ear.

Methods

Having students read relevant chapters in health textbooks is a widely used, traditional method for teaching about hearing health. Since the texts do contain basic curricular information, they can be useful resources when teachers skillfully guide students' reading in them. However, for two reasons at least, instruction should extend beyond texts: (1) to create and provide hands-on activities so children can experience concepts presented in texts, and (2) to provide additional information on hearing health because textbooks tend to sacrifice in-depth exploration of a topic like hearing health in order to cover as many topics as possible. Below is a list of suggested activities and information resources to help elementary school teachers go beyond health texts:

Activities

(1) *Examining an audiogram.* Most or all students have had their hearing tested with an audiometer, but few ever get to see and explore an audiogram, which is a graph of results of an audiometer exam. Studying an audiogram can introduce students to many important concepts, such as sound intensity (measured in dB) and sound frequency (measured in Hertz). When students compare different audiograms they can learn how a hearing impaired person might be able to hear some sounds and not others. A good related activity would be to examine an audiogram of a person with a hearing loss that occurs at selected frequencies and then determine which familiar sounds the subject of the audiogram would be unable to hear.

(2) *Examining headphones, ear plugs, and other hearing protection devices.* Apply the principle of "seeing is believing," or in this case, "hearing is believing." Using a sound effects record or any loud sound source, create an opportunity for every child to experience how ear plugs or other hearing protection devices cut down the volume of sound but still permit the wearer to hear enough to continue functioning safely at the task at hand.

(3) *Keeping a noise log.* To increase students' awareness of sounds, ask them to "just listen" for two minutes or so and write, in a notebook, sources of sounds they hear. Do this activity in the lunch room and outside, at recess; then share results in a discussion. Using a graph of intensities and frequencies of sound sources (watch tick—30dB; air conditioner—60 dB) from the health text or obtained from the Environmental Protection Agency, have students find out the intensities and frequencies of as many sound sources in their noise logs as possible.

(4) *Discovering noise-insulation.* To demonstrate how some materials are better sound insulators than others, drop a marble from the same height onto an empty metal container, a piece of carpet, a floor tile, an acoustic tile, and a piece of wood. Ask students to identify which material deadens the sound most and, as a class, try to explain why. Using their noise logs, children can note use or absence of noise insulating materials throughout the school and in their homes.

(5) *Learning about hearing health professionals.* Students should be aware that noise and hearing loss are serious problems in American society, and that people in many professions work to resolve these problems. One such professional usually is employed in the school system—the speech, hearing, and language professional. Invite this person to share with your class his or her experiences and knowledge of screening and referring persons with hearing impairment as well as of helping children overcome speech and language problems. For different perspectives on hearing health concerns other professionals, such as lawyers, can be invited to explain how laws are written to limit excessive noise

in public places; government officials, to explain how laws are written to limit excessive noise in public places; government officials, to explain how noise-limiting laws are enforced; and construction and faculty managers, to explain what measures management and workers must take to protect their hearing.

Information Resources

Sounds Alive: A Noise Workbook. Donna McCord Dickman, Ph.D., Washington, DC: Metropolitan Washington Council of Governments for U.S. Environmental Protection Agency, Office of Noise Abatement. Available from: E.R.I.C. Document Reproduction Services, P.O. Box 190, Arlington, VA 22210. (703) 841-1212.

Sounds Alive is a handbook of activities for building student awareness of noise and noise pollution control, including games and charts which address the topics of sound measurement, effects of noise on people, methods of noise control, and other related areas.

Sound and Hearing: Understanding the Hearing Impaired. Washington, DC: National Grange, 1981. Available from: National Grange, 1615 H Street, N.W. Washington, DC 20006.

This activities program was designed to teach students in grades 4-5 about sounds, hearing, and deafness. The packet suggests class activities in four areas: ("How Do We Hear?," "How Does Deafness Happen?," "Are Deaf People Different?," and "Total Communication").

NAHSA Hearing Health Classroom Guide and Poster Packet. Rockville, MD. National Association for Hearing and Speech Action. Available from: National Association for Hearing and Speech Action, 10801 Rockville Pike, Rockville, MD 20852. (800) 638-TALK.

A classroom packet which includes a full-size color poster, 25 small coloring posters and a teacher's guide on the themes of protecting one's hearing and awareness of hearing loss. Topics include the role of an audiologist, how to clean one's ears, what to do if one has trouble hearing, the effects of loud noise on hearing, the value of hearing and its effects on children's learning.

CONSUMER HEALTH

DEVELOPING FAST FOOD CONSUMER SKILLS†

Dining in fast food restaurants is a regular part of life for many Americans. On the average, each American eats out almost 200 times a year. Out of every five dollars spent eating out, two dollars go to fast food restaurants (Pruitt & Stein, 1994). Fast food dining often equates to increased fat and sodium consumption and a decrease in nutrient dense and high fiber food choices.

However, fast food restaurants have also provided Americans with convenient access to quick, inexpensive meals that are often a necessity in our sometimes hectic lifestyle. For some subgroups in our culture, such as adolescents, teenagers, and older adults, fast food restaurants have also served as a social center or community meeting place. In some cases the fast food restaurant or shopping mall food court may present the first opportunity for older elementary school children to make their own food choices.

While fast food restaurants continue to offer foods high in fat, sodium, and sugar, many have responded to the increasing nutritional awareness of Americans by adding to or modifying menu selections. Salad bars, fruit juices, low fat/skim milk, whole wheat rolls, and grilled or baked chicken and fish are examples of some of these changes. In many situations it is now possible to order fast food meals with increased nutritional quality.

The following teaching activities are intended to assist intermediate level elementary children in the development of consumer skills related to fast food dining. Prior to participation in all of these activities, it will be important for students to develop a knowledge base related to the nutritional value and fat, sodium, and sugar levels of different foods. Student should also be aware of the health risks associated with poor dietary habits.

Fast Food Feelings

The "Fast Food Feelings" activity provides an opportunity for students to share their thoughts and feelings about fast food restaurants with each other and their teacher. In addition, the activity provides an opportunity for the teacher to not only become familiar with students' feelings but also to gain an awareness of the role fast food restaurants play in the dietary lives of students.

To begin the activity, the "Fast Food Feelings" sheet is distributed to students (See Figure 1). Students are first given a few minutes alone to write out answers to the items on the sheet. Then students share their responses with each other in small groups. The entire class then discusses their responses with the teacher.

Healthy Choices

Often minor changes in food selection, food preparation, or choice of condiments can have an impact on the fat, sodium, or sugar consumed in a fast food meal. The purpose of this activity is to help students develop skills in making these minor changes.

---

†*By David A. Birch, Ph.D., CHES, School of Health Physical Education and Recreation, Indiana University, Bloomington, IN.*

In this activity the children are given a menu sheet with several meals already identified (see Figure 2). From the menu sheet children will make modifications and changes in the foods listed to decrease the fat, sodium, and sugar in the foods. The changes are listed on the bottom of the sheet. Students can make these changes individually or in small groups. Changes can then be discussed with the entire class. It will be important to stress to students that minor changes in a fast food meal can often lead to a considerable reduction in fat, sodium, and/or sugar. Examples of substitutions/changes that students may make, include the following:

- A single hamburger without mayonnaise for the double cheeseburger.
- A grilled chicken or fish sandwich for the fried fish sandwich or fried chicken nuggets.
- A baked potato or salad with low-fat dressing for the french fries.
- Fruit juice, low fat or skim milk for the soda or milkshake.

An alternative or follow-up activity to the Menu Sheet could be the utilization of actual menus from fast food restaurants. Most restaurants will provide nutritional information for their foods. This information could be used in conjunction with the menus.

Fast Food Consumerism

While some fast food restaurants have moved in the direction of more food choices and nutrition labeling, more consumer pressure may lead to even further changes. The following activities are designed to assist in the development of consumer skills that can be applicable to other areas in addition to food consumerism.

- Assign groups of students to write letters to different fast food restaurants asking for nutritional information for foods on their menus. Each group could then report their findings to the entire class. If a fast food restaurant is unwilling to provide the nutritional information then the group could follow the initial letter with a letter to the restaurant's main headquarters asking for the information.

- Select certain items which may be missing from a specific fast food restaurant's menu or an existing item which could be prepared in a more healthful way (grilling or baking instead of frying, skin removed from chicken breast, etc.). Have students begin a letter writing campaign to the restaurant or its headquarters requesting the changes. Discuss the progress of the campaign in class.

Figure 1

FAST FOOD FEELINGS

- My favorite fast food restaurant is . . .

- My favorite food to order at a fast food restaurant is . . .

- I most often eat at fast food restaurants when . . .

- What I like best about eating at a fast food restaurant is . . .

- What I like least about eating at a fast food restaurant is . . .

Figure 2

SAMPLE MENU

#1
Double cheeseburger
Large French Fries
Soft Drink

#2
Fried Fish Sandwich
Onion Rings
Milkshake

#3
Fried Chicken Nuggets
Cheese Fries
Soft Drink

Substitute for one item in each meal to reduce either fat, sodium, or sugar.

Identify a complete fast food meal low in fat, sodium, and sugar.

Fast Food Advertising

Advertisements for fast food restaurants often become well known in the media culture of both children and adults. Seldom do these advertisements tout the nutritional quality of fast foods. For this activity students can create advertisements that promote healthy choices available at fast food restaurants. The advertisements created can be in the form of posters or even videotapes. Students should be encouraged to use variations of slogans or themes that are utilized in actual fast food advertisements. The actual advertisements can be displayed or shown to others in the school or to parents at parent/school functions.

Fast food dining has become a regular event for many people including children. Through the development of specific skills related to fast food dining, individuals can still enjoy the advantages of quick meals while consuming moderate amounts of fat, sodium, and sugar.

Reference

Pruitt, B. E., & Stein, J. J. (1994). *Healthstyles.* Philadelphia: Saunders College Publishing.

AM I REALLY GETTING THE MESSAGE? AN EXERCISE IN CONSUMER AWARENESS†

[This Teaching Idea is presented as a high school/college activity, however, the Editors believe it can be easily adapted for use at the elementary level.]

Since the profit motive is the driving force behind most of the advertising industry, the primary purpose of advertising is to persuade people to purchase products and services. Unfortunately, this frequently translates into creating needs and manipulating the behavior of ill-informed, gullible consumers who are easily misled by unsubstantiated advertising claims. In a one-month survey of American newspapers and magazines, the Food and Drug Administration found 435 questionable ads, over half of which were for weight-loss products (Miller, 1985).

Assessment of messages contained in advertising is a critical aspect of consumer health. Only by being alert, aware, and analytical can consumers determine which claims are legitimate and which are fraudulent or dangerous. It is appropriate to develop these skills in college students because young adults have tremendous purchasing power and frequently are targeted as an audience by advertisers. Students at this level have expressed a special interest in fraudulent health practices (Gaines, 1984).

This class activity was designed for use in high school and college-level classes. The objective was to provide basic information about advertising techniques and strategies and to encourage students to use this knowledge by analyzing selected advertisements in small group discussions.

Class Preparation

One week prior to the lesson, instruct students to clip or photocopy two advertisements to be brought to class on the day of the lesson. Suggest sources such as magazines, newspapers, tabloids,

---

†By M. Dawn Larsen, Assistant Professor of Health Science, Mankato State University, Mankato, MN. This article was previously published in the Journal of Health Education, November/December 1991, 22(6), 363-364.

pamphlets, and promotional fliers. Having them bring two ads will help guard against duplication of ads within groups.

If the class text does not include material on advertising techniques, instructors should provide students with appropriate information. The following information was adapted from Cornacchia and Barrett (1989). This material was presented in a brief lecture and summarized in a handout for students.

Appeal Techniques Used in Advertising

Puffery: Describes item vaguely or generally with subjective opinions, superlatives, or exaggerations, stating no specific facts. Examples: Bayer works wonders; Pepto-Bismol with the famous coating action.

Power words: Use of words that mean little, but get attention. Examples: fights; works harder; improves; natural; enriched; pure; gentle.

Bandwagon: Implication that "everyone is doing it." Examples: People rely on . . .; used in hospitals and labs; used by millions; isn't it time you tried . . .?

Endorsements or testimonials: Claims of effectiveness by physicians, dentists, entertainers, athletes, other celebrities.

Generalizations: Grand statements that actually are vague and say little. Examples: Winning with Anacin; world-proven; many don't get the vitamins they need.

Imagery/visuals: Subliminal persuasion through appeal to emotion. Examples: Effective use of color; beauty of people or environments; contrast, music, and animation (in commercials).

Novelty/mystical aspects: Implication that a new, different, or mysterious ingredient increases effectiveness. Examples: Nature's beauty secret; contains X from Europe; special ingredients.

Slogans, symbols, humor: Special lyrics, phrases, jokes that help you remember the product. Examples: Nothing runs like a Deere; STP is the racer's edge.

Misleading comparisons: Encourage consumers to jump to conclusions. Examples: Contains twice as much; up to 8-hour relief; relieves pain faster; hospitals use Tylenol 18 times more than all other brands.

Rebates/rewards: Financial incentives for purchasing something. Examples: Special rebate for those who act before May 1; free bonus for first 100 customers; second item for only $1 more!

Scientific studies or evidence: Implication that research has shown a product to be superior. Examples: Clinical tests show; created by research scientists; studies have strongly indicated.

Superiority: Implications that a product performs better than all others. Examples: Leading; best; increased; more of; stronger.

Social appeal: Implications that a product makes you more socially acceptable or places you among the elite. Examples: Raise your hand if you're Sure; L'oreal . . . because I'm worth it!

Discussion Formation Small Groups

Randomly assign students to small groups of five or six students each. Have each contribute one ad for group analysis, avoiding duplication where possible. Distribute consumer health worksheets to all group members, instructing students to use them for collective analysis of the ads. Instructors may list advertising techniques on a chalkboard or have students refer to their handouts for assistance in answering question three. This discussion usually takes about 20 or 30 minutes of class time.

Consumer Health Worksheet

1. Explain the "message" the ad is trying to convey (What is your first reaction upon seeing or reading the ad?).
2. To what "part of you" does the ad try to appeal?
   a. Basic needs
   b. Created needs
   c. Values
   d. Emotions

3. What techniques does the ad use to convey the message?
4. What are the suggested consequences of using or not using the product?
5. Does the ad offer evidence to support these claims? If so, is it:
   a. Factual evidence
   b. Scientific verification
   c. Statistical claims
6. Do you feel that the "message" is:
   a. Accurate? Why?
   b. Inaccurate? Why?
   c. Accurate by misleading? Why?
7. Has the ad convinced you to buy the product? How?

If interaction develops slowly, it is helpful for instructors to visit each group to help clarify the assignment and stimulate discussion. Explain that the object of the assignment is not necessarily to achieve consensus but to promote productive and honest discussion of these techniques and their effectiveness. Have students write brief notes and comments about each ad on their consumer worksheets.

Each group should choose one ad to present to the class and one individual to present discussion results. Stress that these should include areas of disagreement as well as consensus. Dissenting opinions may, in fact, be of more interest, since they often lead to animated class discussions. These presentations often overlap into the next class period, since group discussions may have taken 30 minutes of a standard class. If so, give each group a number and have students place their names and group number on their individual consumer worksheets. Instructors then can collect the worksheets and redistribute them by groups during the next class session. This ensures that worksheets will not be lost and minimizes time needed to reorganize groups.

References

Cornacchia, H. J., & Barret, S. (1989). *Consumer health* (4th ed.). St. Louis: Times Mirror/Mosby College Publishing, 68-88.

Gaines, J. (1984). A study of the consumer health interests of selected college students. *Journal of School Health, 54*(11). 437-438.

Miller, R. (1985). Critiquing quack ads. *FDA Consumer, 19,* 10-13.

SUBSTANCE ABUSE PREVENTION

CREATIVE ANTI-SMOKING WARNING LABELS†

Public health authorities suggest the cigarette industry is highly vulnerable to effective counter advertising (Green, 1977). This strategy uses humor to ridicule and debunk the glamorous or macho image of smoking. Few people realize the cigarette industry actually supported legislation to have its advertisements removed from television (Warner, 1985). Cigarette manufacturers did this because their own analysis indicated the "equal time doctrine" mandating a small number of anti-smoking ads on television was having an adverse effect on corporate sales. The cigarette industry supported removal of their ads on television in order to reduce public exposure to effective counter advertising. The cigarette corporations then shifted their television advertising dollars to other methods of advertising such as magazines, point of sale promotion, billboards and sponsorship of music or sporting events. The total number of dollars spent on cigarette promotion last year was 3.27 billion (MMWR, 1990).

The classroom offers a unique opportunity to reuse this highly effective strategy of counter advertising. The following teaching activity has been successfully conducted among fifth and sixth grade students. It also has been used as the basis for a statewide contest.

The objective of the activity is to emphasize the negative social and health liabilities of tobacco use. This is accomplished by having students develop clever rhyming anti-smoking warning labels that could be hypothetically placed on cigarette packages. Negative images of tobacco and humorous, satirical blows to the tobacco industry are encouraged. This teaching activity requires paper, crayons and an overhead projector. Approximately one hour of time is needed to complete the project.

The teacher poses the following question to introduce the topic and test students' knowledge of cigarette warning labels, "What is required by law on all cigarette packages sold in the United States?" Make students aware that the correct answer is no longer a warning label but a series of four rotating warning labels. Have students verbally recall the content of these messages. Use an overhead to briefly review the following actual language of current warnings.

Surgeon General's Warning: Smoking causes lung cancer, heart disease, emphysema, and may complicate pregnancy.

Surgeon General's Warning: Quitting smoking now reduces several risks to your health.

Surgeon General's Warning: Cigarette smoke contains carbon monoxide.

Surgeon General's Warning: Smoking by pregnant women may result in fetal injury, premature birth, and low birth weight.

†By Gordon B. Lindsay, Ph.D., Brigham Young University, Provo, UT; Gary Edwards, M.S., Director, Bureau of Health Promotion and Risk Reduction, Utah Department of Health, Salt Lake City, UT; and Chris Chalkley, M.S., Program Manager, Tobacco Prevention and Control Program, Utah Department of Health, Salt Lake City, UT.

The teacher then states that, while these ads are very accurate, they sound dull and boring. Students are challenged to see who can create the most flashy warning labels to recommend to the Surgeon General. The ads should appeal to youth and focus on short-term immediate consequences of cigarette use. The teacher explains the assignment has the following four rules:

(1) Each label must be four lines long.

(2) The second and fourth lines must rhyme, as in a poem.

(3) The warning must be written on the paper provided by the teacher.

(4) The warning labels should address smoking and not demean smokers.

The teacher sets a completion time and answers questions. Students are provided with a list of tobacco-related words to assist them with the challenge of making the warning labels rhyme. Students should be informed that this list of words associated with smoking is not comprehensive and to use their own ideas.

Potential Words for the Warning Label Contest

smoking	lungs	ill	putrid
smoke	heart	sick	foul
soot	emphysema	butts	nerd
ash	fires	filter	sleazy
pollution	breath	menthol	yucky
tar	doctor	lighter	nausea
nicotine	Surgeon General	ash tray	sports
smell	hospital	matches	athletics
stink	surgery	baby	drug
gross	operation	pregnant	addiction
yellow	death	puff	hooked
teeth	dead	inhale	money
mouth	grave	expire	cost
lips	coffin	stupid	dollar
quit	casket	silly	cents
funeral	price	waste	

Also prime students' creativity by sharing some past examples of rhyming warning labels. The following four are some of the better past entries and do a good job of launching student efforts in the right direction.

Instead of smoking
Go eat a twinkle
You might gain some weight
But you sure won't get stinky.

It hurts little babies
It makes them too small
Advice for young mothers
Is don't smoke at all.

These cigarettes were made
From moldly horse poop.
You're dumb if you smoke them.
Love, Surgeon General Koop

Roses are red
Tobacco is brown.
Athletes don't use it
Cause it slows them down.

After students have submitted their entry, conduct a vote to determine the best anti-smoking messages. Place the ads in a conspicuous place in the school building. Additional coverage of the class activity can be gained by contacting the newspaper, television and radio media to share the more clever entries. Short humorous antidotes are sought for the local news programs. Local radio stations are willing to have students audiotaped reading their warning labels. These short spots can be read at appropriate times such as The Great American Smokeout. Winning ads can be sent to state health departments for wider dissemination. The United States Surgeon General and the United States Office on Smoking and Health would also welcome your students' creativity and correspondence.

Summary

Cigarette counter advertising has been an effective public health education strategy for reducing the number one cause of preventable death in the United States. The promotion of a rhyming warning label contest is a meaningful activity that fosters students' creativity and reinforces the physical, aesthetic and social liabilities of tobacco use. This activity has strong value for media coverage by local newspaper, radio, and television. This teaching technique should be used to complement the important resistance to peer pressure skills training and other necessary components of proven substance abuse curricula.

References

Green, P. (1977). The mass media anti-smoking campaign around the world: Proceedings of the third world conference on smoking and health. PHS DHEW, Pub. No. (NIH) 77-1413.

MMWR. (1990). Cigarette advertising—The United States. *Morbidity, Mortality Weekly Report, 39*(16).

Warner, K. E. (1985). Cigarette advertising and media coverage of smoking and health. *New England Journal of Medicine, 3*(12), 384-388.

DIFFERENT CUPS OF TEA[†]

Teachers have choices. One of the choices they have is how they deliver information. This is not an easy choice. Some ways are easier than others; some ways are more effective than others; some ways are more expensive than others. Think about the following two ways to deliver information about cocaine:

"Describe some of the possible effects of cocaine use on the community."

". . . *increase of violent crime, increase of businesses leaving the community, increase in the number of gangs, and an increase in sickness.*"

That's one way of doing it. Here's another way, from a grades seven-to-nine lesson called Cocaine, in the drug education curriculum *Here's Looking At You, 2000*®, published by Comprehensive Health Education Foundation:

(1) After reading about cocaine and its effects, and after sharing information with classmates, students organize into cooperative learning teams. Each team then gets a work sheet that will enable them to determine how to help a community.

[†]*By Neal Starkman, writer and developer at Comprehensive Education Foundation, Seattle, WA. This article was previously published in the Journal of Health Education, November/December 1993 Supplement, S-47-S48.*

(2) The work sheet describes "The Community," which has seen an increase in use of cocaine and other drugs, particularly among teenagers. The result is that The Community has become less safe and less healthy for the people living in it.

(3) The work sheet describes in detail the people who are threatening The Community: the importers, the gang leaders, the gang members, the "back-up" (young teenagers who serve as lookouts and runners), and the users.

(4) The work sheet describes in detail the people who can help save The Community: police officers, families, school administrators, community groups, and media representatives.

(5) Students draw up a plan to save The Community. The plan must include who will be involved, what they will do, and how they will stop each threat.

(6) Teams then present the plans to the class, and the teacher works with the class to implement at least part of the plans, for example, by selecting someone to speak at a PTA meeting.

Think like an eighth grader: Which class would *you* rather be in? Which class do you think will retain the information longer? Which class do you think will be motivated to learn more?

The point? Lecture and discussion is not every student's cup of tea. Nor is singing. Nor is watching a video. Nor listening to an audio, reading a book, playing a game, doing a role play. But, together, now you've got a curriculum!

Here are a few more examples, based on lessons already developed for curricula like *Here's Looking At You, 2000®*:

Audiotapes

Think about making an audiotape of sounds of activities that kids can take part in instead of taking drugs. Then let students guess what the sounds represent: playing cards, bowling, dancing, swimming. The audiotape is engaging, and it also emphasizes safe, healthy, and fun alternatives to drugs.

Books

In a high school lesson on the AIDS prevention curriculum *Get Real about AIDS™*, published by Comprehensive Health Education Foundation, students read a book called *Your Decision*. The book lets the reader make decisions about relationships, drugs, and sex, select any of dozens of paths based on those decisions, and explore the consequences of those decisions. Interactive books like *Your Decision* help students participate in their *own* stories.

Videotapes

Videotapes are not a magic formula, even though both students and teachers like them. Effective videotapes, like effective books, *engage* the student. Consider videotapes that model skills: The most effective videotapes will be ones in which students can relate to the situations portrayed.

Posters

Ask students to make their own posters, either as a cross-age activity (e.g., middle-school students can make posters for students in lower grades) or for their own classroom. Posters are effective when they're dramatic, concise, and leave a lasting image. They can be used as springboards for discussions as well as closing thoughts.

Board Games

In *Get Real about AIDS™*'s upper elementary and middle school units, a game called Immunity helps students review what they've learned about HIV and AIDS. Students divide into two teams, T-cells and Germs, and plan strategies dependent upon their ability to answer questions. You can have students make up their own board games, too. Think about the objectives of the lesson, and write content cards based on those objectives. Then, students can move various spaces and try to achieve certain goals based on how well they know the information.

Magazines

Here's Looking At You, 2000®'s grades four-through-twelve units feature a magazine made specifically for the curriculum—*Here & Now*™. The magazine gives students information about drugs and chemical dependency by using a student-friendly format that includes jokes, quizzes, stories, interviews, and fun graphics. One advantage of a class making its own magazine is that there's something to do for everyone: writing, graphics, proofreading, research, and coordination.

Plays

In the grades ten-through-twelve unit of *Here's Looking At You, 2000*®, students put on a play called *Lana and Aaron Meet the Just-Say-No Students from Another Galaxy*. In the play, two students try to make an effective decision among many sources of influence. Students love plays; again, it's an engaging way to deliver information.

Conclusion

There are many other cups of tea, all around you. Elementary school teachers, in particular, are known for using the most common items (paper clips, pine cones, poker chips) in order to teach students important concepts. And sometimes a funny thing happens: your work becomes students' play.

Having only one cup of tea is boring and often not very nutritious. Think about the different ways *you* learn. Quite often, in education, the medium is the message. We need to use as many media as we can to get across as many messages as we can.

TIC-TAC-TOE†

Want to get your students interested, involved, and excited? Need something different to motivate everyone from the brightest to the least gifted in your classes? Strike it rich with something as simple as tic-tac-toe.

In tic-tac-toe students pair up and administer their own game by being master/mistress of ceremonies, judge, and contestant at the same time. Students love to compete and cannot be passive while playing this game. It's based on the timeless game everyone knows how to play, so attention can be placed on learning or reviewing the material at hand.

First, I wrote questions and answers on our current unit. Questions were then judged as easy, medium, or difficult. Difficult questions should not be true/false, in order to eliminate guesswork. The number of questions can be adjusted to your material or time restraints. Table 1 lists a sample of questions used in our substance abuse edition.

I began with 25 easy and medium questions and 6 difficult questions. Fewer difficult questions are needed because they earn fewer squares within the tic-tac-toe grid. The questions are typed with the acceptable answers following. For example: Chewing tobacco causes a white patch in the mouth called _____ . (leukoplakia)

One copy of each question is needed for each two students in the class. I used several different methods for preparing the necessary questions. They can be typed on colored paper, coded for the degree of difficulty. Another way is to type all questions on white paper and code them for difficulty by marking the end of the sheets with the appropriate color. One copy of each question is then placed in an envelope; the envelope is sealed and slit at one end to expose the color coded end of the questions (questions can thus be selected without being read). Another method is to print the questions on cardstock, of three different colors; these are more durable but take more time to prepare.

---

†By Mary Lawler, teacher at Greenfield Central High School, Greenfield, IN. This article was previously published in the Journal of Health Education, January/February 1993, 24(1), 58-60.

The class is divided into partners to begin the game. Once a player selects a difficulty level, their opponent reads the appropriate level question from the cardstock stack or envelope. The first player answers and, if correct, places their symbol, X or O, in the tic-tac-toe grid. Xs or Os earned with correct responses to easy questions can only be placed in the four corners, medium questions in the mid-box, and difficult questions in the center of the grid, as shown in Figure 1.

Missed questions are returned to the stack or envelope and remain in play until answered correctly. It is possible the question may recycle to be asked of the player who previously played it. However, it is entirely by chance and students are rewarded for remembering. Only the difficulty of the question is in the control of a player, not the actual question selected.

Players continue taking turns until the game is won or a draw is declared. Players then draw a new tic-tac-toe grid, and continue playing until all questions have been answered correctly and taken out of play. Progress throughout the game varies with ability of the students. Students in my health classes (grades 9 and 10) play the entire packet in 30 to 45 minutes.

Students benefit by working at a self-paced, directed activity at a difficulty level of their own choosing. They are involved on task with reading, answering, judging answers, and planning strategy. The teacher's role should be only as final judge for accuracy and fairness.

The game is easily adaptable to any subject material and grade level. It has been a fun, exciting activity that left my students involved, interested, and excited over health class.

Table 1

QUESTIONS AND ANSWERS
FOR THE SUBSTANCE ABUSE UNIT

Easy Questions

1. Name a drug in the narcotic category. (heroin, codeine, methadone, morphine, opium)
2. What are the narcotics used for in medicine? (stop pain, stop a cough, stop diarrhea)
3. What is the natural source for narcotics? (opium, poppy plant)
4. Where is all cocaine grown? (South America)
5. Free-basing is a method of using which drug? (cocaine)
6. Is caffeine a stimulant? (yes)
7. Can you overdose on caffeine? (yes, but it takes a lot)
8. What effect does a barbiturate have on a person? (can calm or put you to sleep)
9. Do anti-depressants make people high? (no)
10. What group of drugs make a person see things which aren't really there? (hallucinogens)
11. _____ is anything which causes a change in your body physically, mentally, or emotionally). (drug)
12. Stopping drug use and getting sick because the addiction isn't fed is called _____. (withdrawal)
13. _____-dependence involves both tolerance and withdrawal. (physical)

14. _____-dependence means you think you need the drug. (psychological)
15. Name one cancer besides lung cancer caused by tobacco use. (oral, kidney, throat)
16. In 1972 cigarette ads were banned on _____. (TV and radio)
17. _____ is a disease caused by smoking and is both incurable and progressive. (emphysema)
18. Name three things you cannot do while smoking. (answers will vary but may include swim, kiss, live)
19. What type of alcohol is found in alcoholic beverages? (ethyl)
20. What is the only organ in the body which can break down alcohol? (liver)
21. If someone had four mixed drinks, how long would it take to break down all of the alcohol in their body? (four hours)
22. Which produces a stronger beverage: fermentation or distillation? (distillation)
23. What usually happens when the BAC level reaches 10% (death)
24. Which happens first with alcohol use: relaxation or loss of balance? (relaxation)
25. Name the organization which works with teen-agers who live with an alcoholic. (alateen)

Medium Questions

1. What is the disease in which fat replaces normal cells due to the damage done by alcohol? (cirrhosis)
2. What is the best way to quit smoking? (cold turkey)

3. What narcotic is often found in cough medicine and pain relievers? (codeine)

4. Name a medical use for amphetamines. (narcolepsy or hyperactivity)

5. What is the most commonly used drug is America? (alcohol)

6. Approximately __% of all fatal auto accidents involve alcohol. (50)

7. Which drug is the most addictive in the world? (cocaine)

8. What is the term for needing increasing doses of a drug to get the same effect? (tolerance)

9. _____ in tobacco makes it addictive. (nicotine)

10. _____ in tobacco causes cancer. (tar)

11. What group is the only American group to increase its tobacco use? (teenage girls)

12. Which gets into your system faster: a smoked cigarette or chewing tobacco? (smoke)

13. Which has more tar, ammonia, carbon monoxide, and hydrogen cyanide: mainstream or sidestream smoke? (sidestream smoke)

14. Proof is equal to ___ times the percent of alcohol. (two)

15. _____ is when an alcoholic cannot remember. (black-out or alcohol amnesia)

16. _____ oz. of beer has an equal amount of alcohol as _____ oz. of wine. (12:5)

17. Five ounces of _____ has as much alcohol as a shot of _____. (wine:hard liquor)

18. 1 1/2 oz. of whiskey has _____ oz. of ethanol. (1/2)

19. What is the active ingredient in marijuana? (THC or delta-9 tetrahydrocannabinol)

20. One marijuana joint has the same ability to cause cancer as _____ of cigarettes. (one)

21. Name the hallucinogen which causes violent hallucinations and was once used as an anesthetic for animals. (PCP)

22. Most names for prescription depressants end in _____. (-al)

23. When legal penalties have been decreased for drug use or possession it has been _____. (decriminalized)

24. _____ are abused to build muscles and may lead to cancer and other health problems. (steroids)

25. Glue, butyl nitrate, and gasoline belong to the group of drugs known as _____. (inhalants)

Difficult Questions

1. Chewing tobacco causes a pre-cancerous white patch in the mouth called _____. (leukoplakia)

2. Lung cancer is _____% fatal. (95%)

3. The lit end of a cigarette reaches what temperature? (900-1200 degrees F)

4. What would be the effect of 60 milligrams of nicotine taken all at once? (death)

5. What's the difference between a problem drinker and an alcoholic? (alcoholic is addicted, problem drinker's drinking leads to problems but they may not be addicted)

6. _____ is a drug used for aversion therapy in treating alcoholism. (antabuse)

Figure 1

EASY	MEDIUM	EASY
MEDIUM	DIFFICULT	MEDIUM
EASY	MEDIUM	EASY

HEALTH PROMOTION

CREATIVE HEALTH EDUCATION AND THE HEALTHY STUFFED ANIMAL/MUPPET ADVENTURE†

Creativity can be defined in a variety of ways, but one of the most useful ideas is that creativity should be fun. Teachers should not stifle learning and should have as much fun doing creative projects as the students do.

Creativity Learners

Creativity is the rare capacity for developing insights, sensitivities, and appreciations in intellectual or artistic activity. Dorothy Rodgers, a child psychologist, reminds us that different types of learners exist, the bright child and the creative child. Both can have equally high levels of IQ and excellent capacities for learning. The bright child fits well into the traditional structured academic environment. Creative students may not fit the expectation of the teacher and may be labeled as unwilling to cooperate if the teacher fails to recognize their creative aspects (Rodgers, 1969).

Howard Gardner, a Harvard psychologist, takes the creativity learning idea even further and suggests seven differences in learning, or multiple intelligences. The seven intelligences are:

(1) *Linguistic intelligence* is found in students who have highly developed auditory skills and enjoy creative activities with sounds or language.

(2) *Logical/mathematical* learners, being conceptual thinkers, love to manipulate the environment and to expore patterns, relationships, and categories.

(3) *Spatial intelligence* is seen in students who find they do best in seeing things done graphically or in picture form. Spatial learners day dream a lot.

(4) *Musical intelligence* is found in students who like music. These students are sensitive to non-verbal sounds in the environment. They are rhythmically oriented.

(5) The *bodily-kinesthetic* learner is physically active. These kids process knowledge through bodily sensations. Some are gifted with fine motor coordination and do well in sports and physical activities.

(6) *Interpersonal intelligence* students are the people-oriented students. They may be seen emerging as leaders among their peers. These students can organize, manipulate people, socialize, and communicate well with others.

(7) *Intrapersonal intelligence* is seen in children who possess strong personalities. Most shy away from group activities and prefer to bloom in solitude and show a strong sense of independence.

Cone of Learning: Experiential Learning in Health Education

Several educationally related constructs promote creative health education in a school setting. One key construct is that health education should be as experiential as possible. The closer the learning activity can come to providing real meaning to the student, the more likely the learning will

---

†*By Thomas C. Timmreck, Professor in the Department of Health Science and Human Ecology, California State University, San Bernardino, San Bernardino, CA. This article was previously published in the Journal of Health Education, March/April 1994, 25(2), 114-115.*

be retained. If the learning experience can be kept at the bottom of the "Cone of Learning" (Dale, 1954), the more likely it is that it will be experimental (see Figure 1).

One creative way to tap into the different learning styles while providing an experiential approach is to connect school health education activities to health learning at home. One such creative activity is the "Stuffed Animal Health Education Learning Adventure."

The Healthy Stuffed Animal Adventure as a Learning Experience

The healthy stuffed animal adventure is a fun experiential learning activity which causes the elementary student to become involved with assessing his or her own personal health and nutritional behaviors through the medium of a stuffed animal or a muppet-type puppet. The stuffed animal goes home with the child and participates in the same health-related activities that the child does. This creative health education activity allows students with different approaches to learning to experience their own health behaviors while interacting with a stuffed animal or a muppet—a non-threatening friend that all children can relate to. This project works best in the middle levels of elementary school experience. For the "adventure" to be effective, it should be a part of a major unit on health. The children need some understanding about health and nutrition in order for the "adventure" to have its highest level of success.

How the Adventure Works

The elementary teacher obtains a washable 12-inch (or so) stuffed animal such as a rabbit or other cute animal (or muppet-type puppet). All students should have an equal chance of taking the stuffed animal home on its adventure.

The teacher develops a chart system to check the animal out and back in each time. The animal is to go home with the child after school, spending the afternoon, evening, night, and morning with the student and is checked in at the beginning of the school day the next morning. The teacher needs to obtain a large tote bag to put the animal and its personal items in since students take the stuffed animal home on the bus or have to walk and need a way of carrying it.

A journal or log book is needed. The log book goes home with the child, who keeps a running written narrative of the overnight stay. In the running written narrative, the child tells of the fun and adventurous things that happen. Most of all, the written narrative should tell about all the health promoting activities and other related events that occurred while the two of them were together on the overnight adventure. The student should write down whether he or she exercised while playing, what he or she had for snacks, dinner, and breakfast, and about taking a bath, brushing teeth, washing hands (sanitation), sleeping, and other fun activities.

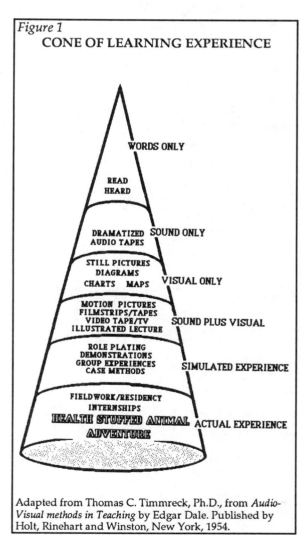

Figure 1
CONE OF LEARNING EXPERIENCE

WORDS ONLY

READ HEARD

DRAMATIZED AUDIO TAPES   SOUND ONLY

STILL PICTURES DIAGRAMS CHARTS MAPS   VISUAL ONLY

MOTION PICTURES FILMSTRIPS/TAPES VIDEO TAPE/TV ILLUSTRATED LECTURE   SOUND PLUS VISUAL

ROLE PLAYING DEMONSTRATIONS GROUP EXPERIENCES CASE METHODS   SIMULATED EXPERIENCE

FIELDWORK/RESIDENCY INTERNSHIPS
HEALTH STUFFED ANIMAL ADVENTURE   ACTUAL EXPERIENCE

Adapted from Thomas C. Timmreck, Ph.D., from *Audio-Visual methods in Teaching* by Edgar Dale. Published by Holt, Rinehart and Winston, New York, 1954.

Students can give the animal small health-promoting gifts if they want (no food items). The child gives a short presentation to the class at the beginning of the next school day on adventures with the stuffed animal. Focus on telling about health promoting activities. The teacher may let the student use the log book to help remember what he or she did on the overnight adventure.

The teacher should write up a set of instructions and rules for the overnight adventure. The instructions should be pasted in front of the log in a manner that will last through the 30 to 40 adventures. Instructions should include care of the animal, carrying and handling the stuffed animal on the bus, how to write in the journal, and what to write in the journal. The teacher may provide a few specific health-promoting activities to look for to record in the journal.

A washable animal should be selected. A muppet-type puppet, if sturdy and cute, might be an even more fun and creative approach. When giving the report, the student could talk through the puppet. Muppet-type puppets can be fun to play with, and they provide much more interaction than a stuffed animal. Another creative approach would be for the teacher to serve as the puppeteer and make the puppet come alive by asking students about the fun and healthy things they did. The teacher could use the log for a prompt to have the puppet converse with students about the overnight adventure. Muppet-type puppets are curious, life-like, and intriguing to all ages and would be welcomed into the home of the student (Timmreck, 1978).

Creative health education is a fun and exciting adventure for the elementary teacher. Learning styles and approaches of students considered, fun learning mediums such as muppet-type puppets and stuffed animals, allow the greatest participation by all students. Experientially based health education adventures are most rewarding for the student because school and learning at home are brought together.

References

Armstrong, T. (1987). *In their own way.* New York: St. Martin's Press.

Dale, E. (1954). *Audio-visual methods.* New York: Holt, Rinehart and Winston.

Gardner, H. (1983). *Frames of mind.* New York: Basic Books.

Greene, W. H., & Simons-Morton, B. G. (1990). *Introduction to health education.* Prospect Heights, IL: Waveland Press.

Rodgers, D. (1969). *Child psychology.* Belmont, CA: Brookes/Cole.

Rubinson, L., & Alles, W. F. (1984). *Health education.* St. Louis: Times Mirror/Mosby.

Timmreck, T. C. (1978). Creative health education through puppetry. *Health Education, 9*(1), 40-41.

JUNIOR HIGH SCHOOL STUDENTS AS FACILITATORS OF ELEMENTARY SCHOOL HEALTH EDUCATION CARNIVALS†

During the early 1980s, Watts and Stinson (1981) began to advocate "health education carnivals" for elementary school students. These carnivals are similar to traditional health education fairs which have been popular for years (Daughtrey, 1976; Lafferty, Guyton & Pratt, 1976; McKenzie, Scheer & Williams, 1981). The most obvious similarity of the carnivals and fairs is that they both employ many of the same instructional strategies and materials. However, where a typical health fair includes

†*By Parris R. Watts, Associate Professor of Health Education at the University of Missouri-Columbia, Columbia, MO, and David K. Hosick, former eighth grade science and health teacher in the Phelps County Missouri School District. He currently is a ninth grade science and health instructor at Blue Springs Junior High School, Blue Springs, MO. This article was previously published in Health Education, October/November 1988, 19(5), 83-85.*

screening tests, the health education carnival does not. The latter actually is comprised of a wide variety of health education activities, incorporated into a festive, carnival-like setting; hence, the reason for its name. Although health professionals still are involved in the carnivals, physicians, dentists and nurses replace their usual work apparel with costumes that are more appropriately related to the activity areas of which they are a part.

Watts and Stinson initially developed the health education carnival concept to expose under-graduate elementary education majors to the natural learning patterns of children prior to a formal student teaching experience. From the beginning, objectives of the health education carnival have been the promotion of (1) personal interaction between the facilitators and children, (2) meaningful health education experiences for the children, (3) cooperative involvement among the facilitators as they plan and implement the activities, and (4) positive public relations within the school and throughout the community. The authors of this article simply have extended those expected out-comes into a new dimension by replacing the elementary education majors with junior high school students. In using junior high school students are facilitators of an elementary school health education carnival, all four of the previously stated objectives were achieved for the elementary students, their school, and the community. Involvement of junior high school students in facilitative roles enabled them to better appreciate their own health within a context of a broader based experi-ence. In addition, they were able to develop a sense of teamwork by joining together in a common cause. Also, the junior high school students were given a great deal of responsibility for providing a quality health education learning opportunity for elementary school students, and they felt much personal pride when their efforts were successful.

Organizing Junior High School Students as Facilitators

The carnival idea was presented to eighth grade students of the Phelps County Missouri School District as a part of their junior high school science and health education course. Video tapes of other carnivals were shown and synopses of certain journal articles were distributed for review (Watts & Stinson, 1981; Petty & Pratt, 1982; Bays, 1986; Wolf, 1986). After students informally discussed the idea among themselves and considered it as a group, they decided to conduct the carnival. It should be noted that the health education carnival was not the only learning activity within the course. A health textbook was utilized and traditional health education class sessions were held throughout the semester. In preparation for the health education carnival, the class was divided into five different groups. After the groups were organized, each was given the opportunity to choose from among five health conceptual areas included in the carnival. Those instructional areas were (1) smoking, alcohol, and other drugs, (2) physical fitness, (3) nutrition, (4) dental health, and (5) first aid. Figure 1 outlines tasks completed by students and by the teacher of the course during the nine weeks devoted to preparation for and staging of the health education carnival event.

Overview of Activity Areas

Following are brief descriptions of the five conceptual areas included in the health education carnival.

Smoking, Alcohol, and Other Drugs—Employed a smoking machine to demonstrate the effects of cigarette smoke on the lungs along with the encouragement not to smoke. Brief descriptions of what happens within the human body when people drink alcohol or use other drugs. Playing of a smoking, alcohol and other drugs game which included basic questions about those substances, with emphasis placed on advantages of not using them. Distribution of coloring books, iron-on and stick-on patches and informational pamphlets pertaining to this activity area.

Physical Fitness—Display of a model of the human heart and identifying and explaining its vari-ous anatomical parts. Use of a stethoscope for students to listen to their heartbeats and to participate in a physical activity and then listen to determine how much faster their hearts beat in response to exercise. Playing of a game which emphasized the sequence of blood flow through the chambers of the heart and reviewed how the heart works. Distribution of pamphlets and other resource materials on blood circulation and the benefits of maintaining physical fitness throughout the elementary school years and beyond.

```
┌─────────────────────────────────────────────────────────────────────────────────────┐
│ Figure 1                                                                              │
│                  STUDENT TASK ASSIGNMENTS AND TEACHER CHECKLIST                        │
│                                                                                       │
│ Weeks                           Student Task Assignments                              │
│                                                                                       │
│ 1-2    Develop the activity/conceptual area, including the selection of a carnival    │
│        theme and send for and/or locally secure information and resource materials.   │
│ 3-5    Organize information received and materials secured for use in the carnival    │
│        activity areas.                                                                │
│ 6-7    Work on banners, posters, handouts, and costuming for the activity areas.      │
│ 8      Complete all preparatory work and rehearse presentations to be made within     │
│        each activity area during the carnival.                                        │
│ 9      Conduct the health education carnival for the elementary school students.      │
│                                                                                       │
│ Weeks                              Teacher Checklist                                   │
│                                                                                       │
│ 1-3    Motivate the junior high school students and offer ideas which will, in turn,  │
│        generate additional ones.                                                      │
│ 4      Start to promote the carnival among the administration, faculty, and staff of  │
│        the school and keep students on task.                                          │
│ 5      Secure volunteers from among school personnel to help publicize the carnival   │
│        within the elementary school and throughout the community (to promote          │
│        parental and family involvement) and continue to keep the students             │
│        progressing in their work.                                                     │
│ 6-7    Encourage carnival facilitators (students) to finalize work on their activity  │
│        areas.                                                                          │
│ 8      Preside over the rehearsal sessions; select student facilitators to visit the  │
│        elementary school classes to promote the carnival event, and make certain that │
│        media coverage is arranged.                                                    │
│ 9      Coordinate the efforts of the student facilitators during the carnival.        │
└─────────────────────────────────────────────────────────────────────────────────────┘
```

Nutrition—Introduction of the four basic food groups and an explanation of the importance of each. Discussion of "junk foods" and provision of actual substitute foods for the children to eat selected from among the four basic food groups. Playing of a nutrition game wherein students reached into a sack of groceries and placed the food item withdrawn into its proper basic food group.

Dental Health—Presentation of a skit involving the elementary students themselves where they were introduced to dental caries and given a graham cracker to eat. Plaque revealed on their teeth and cleansed away by using carrot and celery sticks to demonstrate how foods can help clean the teeth. Proper brushing of the teeth included in the skit, along with other dental hygiene practices.

First Aid—Introduction to the three degrees of burns and a demonstration on how to properly treat each. The correct way to bandage burn injuries in order to help relieve pain and prevent infection stressed. Printed resource materials dealing with burns distributed.

Conducting the Carnival

During the week of the health education carnival, regularly scheduled daily class periods for the eighth grade science and health course on Tuesday, Wednesday, and Friday were used for the carnival. On each of those days, the 56-minute scheduled class time was used to set up, conduct the carnival, and disassemble the activity areas. The first ten minutes of the class period were used to assemble and organize the five activity areas. Then on each day, a different class (second grade on Tuesday, third grade on Wednesday, and fourth grade on Friday) participated in the carnival, held in the school gymnasium. Students in each class were divided into five separate groups and assigned to begin at a different learning center. They were then rotated through all five activity areas so that every student was exposed to each set of learning experiences.

All five groups of junior high school facilitators were given seven minutes to conduct their activity area session. The seven minute time period typically consisted of one minute to introduce to the conceptual material, two minutes of information sharing, two to three minutes of games or other hands-on activities for the children, and one minute to synthesize and conclude the learning experience. During the weeks of preparation for the carnival, the junior high school student facilitators were instructed to design the activity areas so that they would (1) be child-centered, (2) provide basic information at the proper grade level, and (3) promote learning and fun throughout the experience. All three goals were effectively achieved, best evidenced in the attentive behavior and enthusiastic response of the elementary school children.

After all groups had rotated through each station, plenty of time remained for disassembly of activity areas and clearing out of the gymnasium. With everyone working together, there was no need for junior high school students to miss any additional class time outside the regularly assigned science and health class period.

Carnival Follow-Up

After the health education carnival was over, the primary author of this article, who also was instructor of the eighth grade health class, visited elementary school classes involved in the experience. He found students studying, completing the worksheets, and using the pamphlets and other printed resource materials provided for them during the carnival. Elementary school students clearly seemed to be more conscious of their health and expressed considerable interest in following good health habits they had learned during the carnival. Two examples of the lasting impact of the carnival on their lives were noted by the junior high school science and health teacher. Members of the third grade class confessed they had no idea that milk was so good for the body and they proclaimed that they would continue to drink more of it. Members of the second grade class organized a "Smoke Busters" club and promised to wear their "Don't Smoke" emblems to further demonstrate their commitment. The teacher observed that the second grade students remained true to their promise.

Additional follow-up was also done by teachers in each of the three classes involved in the health education carnival. During the next few class meetings, they processed the health related information and materials given to their students. Elementary school teachers expressed sincere appreciation for the outstanding, active learning opportunity made available to their students during the health education carnival. Teachers were surprised that the junior high school students could be so well organized, motivated, and capable of providing such a high quality learning experience for their students. What was possibly even more amazing is that we never doubted for a moment that they could do it. Junior high school students are "naturals" as facilitators of elementary school health education carnivals. Give them the chance and you will be glad that you did!

References

Bays, C. T. (1986). The elementary school health fair: A process involving the whole school in health education. *Journal of School Health, 56*, 292-293.

Daughtrey, G. (1976). The Norfolk public schools health fair. *Health Education, 7*(4), 36-37.

Lafferty, J., Guyton, R., & Pratt, L .E. (1976). The University of Arkansas health fair as professional preparation. *Health Education, 7*(4), 24-25.

McKenzie, J. F., Scheer, J., & Williams, I. C. (1981). The health and safety fair: A cookbook approach. *Health Education, 12*(1), 27-29.

Petty, R., & Pratt, C. (1983). Student staffed health fairs for older adults. *Health Education, 14*(2), 40-42.

Watts, P. R., & Stinson, W. J. (1981). The health education carnival: Giving the old health fair a facelift. *Health Education, 12*(6), 23-25.

Wolf, Z. R. (1986). A health fair for school-age children presented by registered nurses. *Journal of School Health, 56*, 192-193.

MAKE UP YOUR MIND DAY, NATIONAL OATMEAL MONTH, AND OTHER OPPORTUNITIES TO CAPITALIZE ON ANNUAL EVENTS AS A HEALTH EDUCATION STRATEGY†

As far back as the 1850s, when Massachusetts became the first state to mandate the teaching of hygiene in its public schools, health educators have recognized the value of capitalizing on annual events as a strategy for focusing student, parent, and community attention on important health issues of the day. May Day–Child Health Day, inaugurated by Herbert Hoover in 1928 when he was serving as President of the American Child Health Association (Ingen, 1935), and the Summer Round-Up Campaign of the 1920s, which focused on the importance of health examinations for school children (Means, 1962), are two early examples of annual health promotion events.

More recently, school and community health educators have utilized World Health Day, April 7, as an opportunity to share information and experiences related to health conditions worldwide. (World Health Day Planning Kit, 1991). The AAWH also initiated World AIDS Day (December 1) in 1988. Now an annual event in most countries, World AIDS Day encourages increased awareness about HIV infection, supports AIDS prevention and control activities, and promotes support and care for all HIV-infected people (World AIDS Day Action Kit, 1990). Action planning kits, including a resource list and a directory of state contact persons, as well as suggested health education activities, are available for both World Health Day and World AIDS Day.

The plethora of days, weeks, and months has grown, over the years, to the point where, for almost any given day, a health related annual event, presidential proclamation, anniversary, or celebration can be identified. The focuses of many such annual events offer opportunities for linkages to content areas currently included in the scope of comprehensive health education. A few intriguing examples, along with possible linkages, include: Make Up Your Mind Day (decisionmaking), Sorry Charlie Day, a day, named for Charlie Tuna, to recognize anyone who has been rejected (self-esteem), National Oatmeal Month (nutrition), National Joygerm Day, a day for hugging, smiling, grinning, and winning over grumps and grouches (mental health), Week of the Ocean (environmental health), and Cable TV Month (sexuality or physical fitness).

Health educators might use suggestions for classroom activities provided in the event sponsor's promotional material, or ask colleagues and students to brainstorm ways to capitalize on a given annual event. (A healthy measure of skepticism may be in order in the case of some commercial sponsors wherein the sponsor's own agenda for product promotion may not match the health education message desired.)

Some events, Cable TV month for example, may usher in annual health education strategies which are far different from those the sponsor had in mind, but which serve the health educator's purposes rather nicely. Guiding students in an examination of the relationship between what they see on MTV and current teen sexual behavior, or challenging students and their families to live without television for a week and engage in more healthful recreational activities instead, are a few examples.

A variety of learner-centered strategies can be employed to capitalize on annual events. Special programs, photo displays, classroom visitors, student initiated investigations, interviews and research projects, poster contests, classroom discussions, and role plays are all methods for conveying timely messages and promoting healthful behaviors.

Inventing an original annual event, to focus attention on a local concern, or to acknowledge the contribution of a local historical figure to the health education scene is yet another possibility. Local mayors, governors, and other governmental officials often are willing to legitimize an annual event by making an official declaration.

At the federal level, a congressional process, beginning with introduction of a bill in the House or Senate, has been established for declaring special observances. The first presidential proclamation

†By Susan J. Koch, Assistant Professor of Health Education, The University of Northern Iowa, Cedar Fall, IA. This article was previously published in Journal of Health Education, March/April, 1993, 24(2), 113-115.

was made by George Washington when he declared November 26, 1789 Thanksgiving Day, and there have been 6,013 presidential proclamations to date (Chase & Chase, 1990). Contacting a U.S. Senator or Representative who has an interest in the particular health issue is an appropriate way to initiate the presidential proclamation process.

The following steps, adapted from the World AIDS Day action Kit provided by the American Association for World Health, are recommended for planning an annual event:

1. Identify persons/organizations within the school and community who share your interest in observing the event. (This is a good opportunity to establish helpful linkages between schools and community groups.)

2. Form a planning committee representative of interested persons/groups.

3. Brainstorm and select appropriate activities. (Remember to include students in the planning process.)

4. Set a date for your activities—usually dependent upon the official observance date.

5. Make a list of resources needed (personnel, money, supplies, time, etc., and brainstorm about how to access these resources).

6. Determine who is your target audience, that is, who needs to receive this health education message. Discuss ways to get your target audience involved.

7. Make a planning timetable. Schedule dates and deadlines for preliminary preparations and activities from the first planning meeting through the event follow-up.

8. Contact the media and organize publicity. (Decide which media is most appropriate for your event and prepare a press release.)

9. Secure necessary authorizations from school administration and/or other officials.

10. After the event, evaluate the impact of your efforts and thank all who participated. Plan for next year! (World AIDS Day Action Kit, 1990).

There are numerous opportunities for incorporating special events into the health education curriculum (see Figure 1). Capitalizing on annual events as a health education strategy can enliven the health education experience for students, provide healthful opportunities for community-school interaction and service, and engender positive publicity for the school health education program.

References

Chase, W. D., & Chase, H. M. (1990). *Chase's annual events.* Chicago: Contemporary Books.

Means, R. K. (1962). *A history of health education in the United States.* Philadelphia: Lea and Febiger.

Van Ingen, P. (1935). The story of the American Child Health Association. *Child Health Bulletin,* September/November, 29-30.

World AIDS Day Action Kit. (1990). American Association for World Health, Washington, DC.

World Health Day Planning Kit. (1991). American Association for World Health, Washington, DC.

Figure 1

HEALTH RELATED ANNUAL EVENTS

Date	Title	Contact
Sept. 1-30	All American Breakfast Month	The Breakfast Partners, 5770 N. Meridian Indianapolis, IN 46208
Sept. 23	National Good Neighbor Day	Good Neighbor Day Foundation Box 379, Lakeside, MT 59922
Oct. 1-31	National Family Sexuality Education Month	Planned Parenthood Federation of America 810 Seventh Ave., New York, NY 10019
Oct. 25-31*	Peace, Friendship & Goodwill Week	Intl. Society of Friendship & Goodwill Box 2637, Gastonia, NC 28053-2637
Oct. 16	United Nations World Food Day	United Nations Dept. of Public Information New York, NY 10017
Nov. 1-30	Child Safety & Protection	National PTA, 700 N. Rush St., Chicago, IL
Nov. 15	Great American Smokeout (encourages smokers to kick the habit for at least 24 hours)	American Cancer Society, 1180 Ave. of Americas New York, NY 10036
Dec. 1-31	Universal Human Rights Month	Intl. Society of Friendship & Goodwill Box 2637, Gastonia, NC 28053-2637
Dec. 16-22*	Tell Someone They're Doing A Good Job Week	Radio Station WCMS 900 Commonwealth Place, Virginia Beach, VA 23464
Jan. 1-31	National Oatmeal Month	Quaker Oaks Company
Jan. 14-20*	National Pizza Week	Pizza Hut Public Affairs 9111 East Douglas, Wichita, KS 67207
Jan. 8	National Joygerm Day (a day for celebrating joy)	Joygerms Unlimited Box 219 Eastwood Station, Syracuse, NY 13206
Feb. 1-28	American Heart Month	American Heart Association 7320 Greenville Ave., Dallas, TX 75231
Feb. 5-9*	National School Counseling Week	American School Counselor Association 5999 Stevenson Ave., Alexandria, VA 22304
Feb. 3	Elizabeth Blackwell birth Anniversary. 1821 (first U.S. woman physician)	No contact
March 1-31	National Nutrition Month	American Dietetic Association 216 W. Jackson Blvd., Ste 800, Chicago, IL 60606
March 12-18*	American Chocolate Week	Chocolate Mfrs. Association of USA 450 Park Ave. S., New York, NY 10016
March 21	National Teenager's Day	National Teenager's Day 14200 Ventura Blvd. Ste. 106, Sherman Oaks, CA 91423
April 1-30	National Humor Month	Larry Wilde, Bantam Books 660 5th Ave., New York, NY 10103
April 24-30*	National Youth Fitness Week	Athletic X-Press. Dawn Danker-Rosen 233 Broadway, 4th Fl., New York, NY 10279
April 22	Sorry Charlie Day (day to recognize anyone who has been rejected and kept his spunk)	"Sorry Charlie. No-Fan-Club-For-You Club" Cathy Runyan 201 Main Place, Parkville, MO 64152
May 1-31	Mental Health Month	National Mental Health Association
May 7-13*	Clean Air Week	American Lung Association 1740 Broadway, New York, NY 10019-4374
May 1	Student Counselors Day (tribute to peer helpers)	Union Memorial Hospital School of Nursing 201 E. University Parkway, Baltimore, MD 21218

*Exact dates will vary from one year to the next.

IDEAS FOR A SCHOOL HEALTH CLUB†

Many schools both elementary and secondary allot time during the school day and after school for student clubs. Photography clubs, drama clubs, and science clubs are but a few of the more common student clubs found in the school setting. A health club can be another worthwhile student experience to add to a school's extracurricular program.

The formation of a health club for students cannot only provide meaningful health education experiences for the students involved, but also facilitate school-community interaction, promote a healthy lifestyle, and showcase the benefits of a school health education program. Health clubs can provide enrichment to a comprehensive, sequential school health education program that should never take the place of any component of such a program.

Enrichment to a health education program can be provided in several ways. On the secondary level, students are not always offered a health education course at every grade level. Even in situations where health education electives are offered, an interested student may not be able to schedule an elective health education course because of other scheduling demands. For these students the health club can provide health education experiences.

Further study of topics covered in health education classes can provide another opportunity for enrichment. An example of this may be a student who, after studying cardiovascular health in health education class, may conduct further research on the topic resulting in some type of report, project, or field trip. Even when a quality health education program exists, logistical factors can prevent such time consuming activities as field trips, service projects, research projects, organizing and participating in health fairs, and specialized training (CPR, First Aid). All these activities could be considered by a health club.

For the school health educator interested in organizing a health club, the following considerations should be addressed.

(1) Will the sponsor have adequate time for planning club meetings and activities?

(2) Will there be a limit on membership? Will it be open to all grades or only students at certain grade levels? Will there be any eligibility criteria? (Some schools/clubs require students to meet certain academic requirements such as a certain grade point average.)

(3) What will the process be for selecting club activities? What is the best mechanism for providing input of members?

(4) Will the school provide any financial support if needed? Will there be a need for fundraising activities?

(5) Are there volunteers for activities such as field trips when other adults are needed for supervision and transportation?

If, after consideration of these issues, the health educator is ready to proceed, there are many possible activities for a club to undertake The following are some possibilities:

Health Fairs: A club could organize a health fair using community resources for screening, demonstrations, and activities. Club projects could be displayed. In addition to organizing their own health fair, students can be involved in health fairs organized by other groups. Involvement in health fairs organized by other groups could mean the development of an exhibit or audio-visual resources, volunteering for fair duties or club fundraising. Specific ideas for health fairs have been offered in previous editions of *Health Education* (McKenzie et al., 1981; Germer & Price, 1981; Watts & Stinson, 1981).

Assembly Presentations: Club members can give presentations on various health related topics to school assemblies, PTA groups, and other civic and community groups.

Field Trips: Club field trips can be taken to community health facilities including fitness centers, hospitals, clinics, and museums. Follow-up activities to such trips such as picture reports, presentations to other students, and club discussions should be scheduled. Careful planning and specific guidelines are essentials for any field trip (Price, 1978).

---

†*By David A. Birch, Ph.D., CHES, School of Health Physical Education and Recreation, Indiana University, Bloomington, IN. This article was previously published in Health Education, April/May 1986, 17(2), 50-51*

Health News: There are a variety of ways health club members can provide health news to students and others in the community. Most schools have school newspapers and a PA system. A regular health column in the school newspaper and a daily or weekly health message over the PA system can provide a regular service to students. A regular column in the community newspaper can reach community members. A more ambitious project could be the publication of a periodic health newsletter. Using a video cassette recorder and camera, a health news broadcast could be produced and presented to other students.

Debates and Discussions: Debates, panel discussions, or individual presentations on health topics could be organized. These programs could include club members, other students, health professionals, school staff, and community members. Attendance may be limited to club members or may be opened up to other groups.

Fundraising Projects: Fundraising projects could be organized to benefit the club itself or other health related organizations. Club members and the sponsor should keep in mind that a health club should select fundraising activities that promote healthful behaviors, i.e., fun runs, road races, walkathons, and nutritious snack recipe books instead of candy sales or bake sales.

Community Service Projects: Club members can be involved in volunteer projects that promote school and community health. Examples of community service projects are volunteer work in a hospital, community health center, or school health clinic, involvement in community fundraisers, and participation in nursing home activities.

Peer Teaching: In areas of individual interest and expertise, students could be trained to present mini-lessons to club members, other students, and possibly staff or community members. Trained club members could work with small groups of students in the regular health education classroom setting.

Current Health Issues: The health club can provide members an opportunity to examine, discuss or debate current health issues or participate in activities not included in the health education instructional program. Examples of current issues may be new developments in medical technology and the related ethical issues or health-related political issues. Members may want to pursue individual or group research projects related to those issues. Activities such as health-related computer use or the production of health-related videocassettes could be health club ideas. Time or scheduling considerations may prevent participation in these types of activities in the health education instructional process.

Health Education Resource Center: If space can be found, club members may want to organize a health education resource center for other students and possibly community members. There are numerous sources of free or inexpensive health materials that can be collected by club members. Voluntary health agencies, health-related professional agencies, and other health interest groups may be willing to donate resources. The school or community library may be willing to periodically loan materials for resource room use.

Display Case/Bulletin Board: Most schools maintain display cases and bulletin boards in halls, foyers and other common areas. Many times those responsible for maintaining these displays are more than willing to have someone assume responsibility for one or more. Health club members could assume responsibility for periodic bulletin board displays related to health.

With creativity and careful planning, the possible activities for a school health club are limitless. Through such activities, interested students can extend and enrich their health education experiences and possibly expand the health education and health promotion opportunities for other students, school staff, and community members.

References

Germer, P., & Price, J. H. (1981, February). Organization and evaluation of health fairs. *The Journal of School Health,* 86-90.

McKenzie, J. F., Scheer, J., & Williams, I. C. (1981, January/February). The health and safety fair: A cookbook approach. *Health Education,* 27-29.

Price, J. H. (1978, May/June). Field trips. *Health Education,* 43.

Watts, P. R., & Stinson, W. J. (1981, November/December). The health education carnival. *Health Education,* 23-25.

CREATING COMMUNITY WELLNESS BY EMPOWERING MIDDLE SCHOOL PEERS†

The work of David Hawkins and Richard Catalano on risk factor reduction and the research done by Jeanne Gibbs and Sherrin Bennett on protective factors point to the importance of educational efforts structured around cooperative learning, social skills that enhance a sense of personal power and competence, and involvement by youth in prosocial activities with peers and in the community at large. This teaching idea illustrates an approach that can help build bridges between youth and between young people and the larger community, bridges that reduce risk factors, encourage resiliency, empower youth, and contribute to community wellness.

Building Bridges

One especially effective activity to create bonds among students is called "Headbands." Start the activity by asking the group what it means to label other people and what effects labels have on people at school. Following a brief discussion based on these questions, offer a personal example of being labeled. This should be followed by your stating the purpose of the activity: to explore how we label, why we label, and the effects labeling has on both the labeler and the person being labeled. Explain to students that you're going to conduct a role play illustrating the effects of labeling.

Ask for eight volunteers to play the members of a school committee; you play the role of the principal. To set up the role play, ask each of the role players to put on a headband onto which a label can be fastened. Then describe the task of the committee as organizing a school dance where students need to determine, on a minimal budget, the following: the refreshments, the entertainment, and the place, date, and time.

Assign labels to each role player, and be sure that none of the participants can see their own labels. Here are the labels:

Bully: Fear me.
Brain: Compliment me.
Nerd: Make fun of me.
Druggie: Ignore me.
Teacher's Pet: Resent me.
Jock: Tolerate me.
Leader: Follow me.
Clown: Laugh at me.

If these labels are not realistic for your school community, substitute labels that are. Take care that no one receives a label that actually describes that person's subgroup or how that person is treated. Before beginning the role play, encourage the players to speak up and not to be afraid to treat each other as it says they should be treated on their labels, without giving away what the label actually says. Also, let the players know that you will stop the action from time to time as necessary to keep the discussion going.

Reiterate the committee's task to organize the school dance while reacting to each other based more on what the label instructs than on the merit of the idea. The rest of the group will only observe during the role play, but participate in the discussion that follows. The role play should last about 10 minutes.

After the role play has generated a lively exchange, consider the following key discussion questions addressed first to each role player individually:

1. How did it feel being on this committee?
2. Would you want to continue to be on this committee? Why or why not?

†By Kelley Reid, Natural Helpers® Program Coordinator at Comprehensive Health Education Foundation, Seattle, WA. This article was previously published in Journal of Health Education, November/December 1993 Supplement, S-52-S-53.

3. What do you think your label says?

4. Stepping out of your role, is there anything you want to say to anyone in the role play group?

Have all the role players in turn take off their labels and headbands, state their names, and say something they enjoy doing in their free time.

Next, address the following questions to the entire group:

1. What did you notice about how people treated each other in the role play?

2. How did this affect individuals? How did this affect the role-play group?

3. How did labels affect the ability of the group to accomplish its task?

4. How do people get labeled at school?

5. How does this affect the labeler, the person labeled, and the school community?

You may want to break into small groups, then have a large group conduct a final debriefing on Questions 4 and 5 to make it easier for people to open up.

Finally, conclude by restating the purpose of the activity and the importance of being both genuinely ourselves and accepting of others if we are to get along with others and if we want to create a more caring school community.

Conclusion

Creating community wellness means empowering youth to lead us into the future. And, according to researcher Bonnie Benard, there is nothing more important in creating healthy communities than teaching young people the skills they need to "create supportive, nurturing environments that will, in turn, discourage alcohol and drug abuse and other interrelated social problems." Benard goes on to say that "no better preventionist training exists than peer collaboration in mutual problem solving in a climate of mutual helping and respect."

As Morton Deutsch, a seminar researcher in conflict resolution, has said, "It has been increasingly recognized in recent years that our schools have to change in basic ways if we are to educate children beyond hate so that they are for rather than against one another." The "Headbands" activity described here is one piece of what needs to be a comprehensive approach to giving students the skills they need to build bridges and create nurturing environments.

The "Headbands" activity described in this article was developed by C.H.E.F.® for its Natural Helpers® program. For more information on Natural Helpers®, call Kelley Reid at 1/800/323-2433.

For more information on Jeanne Gibbs's and Sherrin Bennett's protective factors research, contact them at Interactive Learning Systems, 1505 Bridgeway, Suite 121, Sausalito, CA 94965, (415) 331-4073.

For more information on David Hawkins's and Richard Catalano's risk factor research, contact them at Developmental Research and Programs, Inc., 130 Nickerson, Suite 107, Seattle, WA 98109, (206) 286-1805.

References

Benard, B. (1991). The case for peers. *The Peer Facilitator Quarterly, 8*(4), 20-27.

Deutsch, M. (1989, March 19). *Educating beyond hate.* Paper presented for Elie Wiesel Conference on the Anatomy of Hate. Boston University.

ACROSS THE CURRICULUM

Developing a physical education curriculum that integrates the seven levels of intelligences is a challenge. This latest theory of teaching currently influencing curriculum development involves a new approach not only in the classroom but also in physical education.

The theory of the multiple intelligences developed by Harvard's Howard Gardner, in his book *Frames of Mind: The Theory of Multiple Intelligence,* presents at least seven human intelligences. The two most common intelligences are verbal/linguistic and logical/mathematical. These two areas are emphasized in schools. The other five intelligences, spatial, musical, kinesthetic, interpersonal and intrapersonal, have not been given high priority in the academic setting.

Gardner arrived at this theory of the seven levels of intelligences through his extensive research of studying children of all cultures and ages. A brief summary of the seven levels is:

- Linguistic intelligence learns through the written word
- Logical-mathematical intelligence learns through the ability to think mathematically
- Bodily-kinesthetic intelligence learns through movement
- Spatial/Visual intelligence learns through space and visual representations
- Musical intelligence learns through beat, melody, rhythm
- Interpersonal intelligence learns through working with others
- Intrapersonal intelligence learns through knowing himself/herself.

Traditional techniques of teaching don't always reach every child. Different learning styles need creative approaches to education. An active hands-on approach can reach those students who need a non-traditional approach to education. This approach of including the seven levels of intelligences combined with integration to the curriculum is a basic and necessary part of a complete education spectrum.

Teaching traditional movement and sport activities is a standard approach to educating the young child in physical education. This technique, while teaching motor development and games, does not integrate with educational themes nor does it incorporate all levels of intelligences. This concept of combining the multiple intelligences theory of Howard Gardner's plus academic integration inspired "Moving Young Minds."

The following lesson is designed for the young learner and is a physical education lesson. It follows a lesson on ecology. The whole lesson can be adapted for a classroom.

Basic Integration Theme:	Earth Day
Basic Movement Objective:	Stretching, push-ups, marching, sit-ups, hopping, running, skipping
Basic Intelligence:	Kinesthetic, Linguistic
Objective:	Musical/rhythmic. Interpersonal

---

†*By Sally Smith, Elementary Physical Education Specialist, Purdy Elementary School, Gig Harbor, WA.*

Equipment:	Tape recorder, music, posters of garbage, signs for warm-ups, 4-5 hula hoops, 4-5 nerf balls, 2-4 jerseys
Safety:	Stress to students to watch where they are going
Introductory Activity:	Linguistic intelligence

WALL CHANGE

Place acid rain poster, oil spill poster, recyclable objects, and garbage on different walls of the gym. Instruct the students to perform specific stretches while facing the different walls.

Recyclable: Turn to a wall that shows items that we can recycle. While you are thinking about ways you can separate your recyclables in your house and at school, do a stretch for the back of your legs.

Garbage: Turn to the wall that shows garbage that will be on our earth for the next 100 years. While you are thinking about ways you can stop using these products, do a stretch for the front of your legs.

Acid Rain: Turn to the wall that shows the effects of acid rain. While you are thinking about the animals and plants that are harmed by these chemicals and pollutants in the rain, do a good stretch for the lower back.

Oil Spill: Turn to the wall that shows the effects of an oil spill. While thinking about the effects of black oil on our fish and birds, do a stretch for your arms.

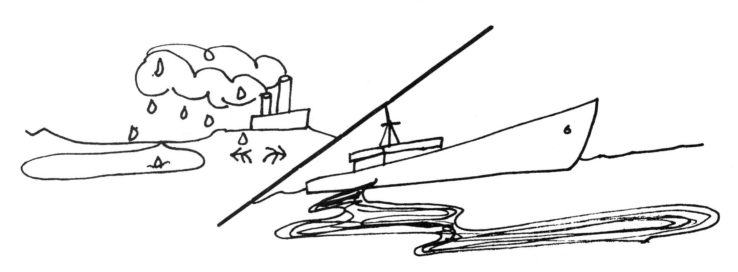

Warm Ups: Linguistic Intelligence

EARTH DAY CHANT

Signs made with Earth Day slogans and exercises. Make slogans on red paper for students to stop and read, green paper for exercises.

Arrange class in scattered formation. Randomly hold signs up for all to read and follow the commands. For younger students, use the pictures provided and enlarge to fit on posters. Space signs to ensure that exercises are performed properly. Allow time for students to work on fitness through repetition of exercises.

Sign Suggestions:

RED	GREEN
Save Our Earth	Do sit-ups; show your worth
Give Paper and Bottles Back	Do some jumping jacks
Don't Throw Junk Away	Do push-ups here today
Recycling Cans Is Fun	Everyone run
Save Water; Don't Let it Drip	Go for a skip
Protect the Layer of Ozone	March around on your own
Oil Spills Must Stop	In place, everybody hop
Plant a Shrub or Tree	On your back, squeeze your knees

Lesson: Bodily/Kinesthetic Intelligence and Interpersonal Recycling Machine

Divide the class into four to six groups. Each group will have a recycling problem. The goal of the assignment is to develop a machine that can be used to help solve this problem. The machine must be made by using students' bodies as parts. Does your machine have any movable parts? Does your machine make noise? Do all parts work at once? Allow creative time for class to work on creations. Once all machines are designed, have each group present its project. The following are suggestions for group projects: litter, plastic recycling, paper recycling, oil spill clean-up machine, acid rain clean-up machine.

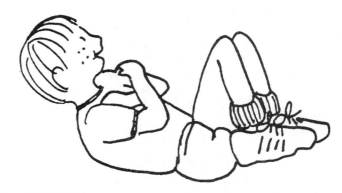

SIT-UPS

Game: Bodily/Kinesthetic Intelligence

Exxon Valdez

Area: Gym, playground

Equipment: 4-5 hula hoops, 4-5 nerf balls, 2-4 jerseys

Players: Class, kindergarten-5th grade

On the whistle, Exxon Valdez (taggers) run to Spill Oil (tag) the fish who are the runners. Once tagged, player must freeze. He/she then must plead to a Clean-up Crew Member "Help," the closest Clean-up Crew Member throws the ball. If the player catches it, he/she is free (must return the ball to the Clean-up Crew Member). The Clean-up Crew Member must go get the ball if the frozen player fails to catch it. After 2-3 minutes, the whistle blows and players, Exxon Valdez and Clean-up Crew Members switch. Fish (runners) may not all be able to switch.

Variations: Grades 3, 4, 5 must throw and catch the ball from the Clean-up Crew Member. Grades K, 1, 2 can bounce or roll.

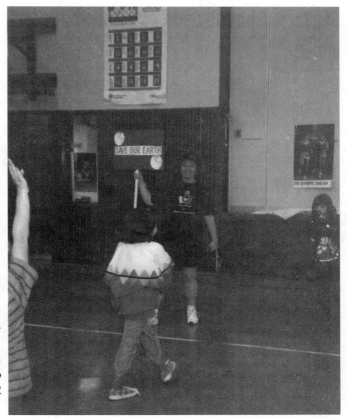

Closure: Musical Intelligence

Earth Day Rap

Turn up the volume
The time is now
To save our earth
Make a difference somehow.

Arrange class in scattered formation. Practice the chant. Repeat chant three times, increase the volume with each repeat.

Suggested Records:

"Hug the Earth," Tickle Tune Typhoon, P.O. Box 15153, Seattle, WA 98115
"Wecology," Friends Around the World, Jim Valley, Rainbow Planet, 5110 Cromwell Drive, Gig Harbor, WA 98335

References:

Dauer, V., & Pangrazi, R. (1983). *Dynamic physical education for elementary children.* Burgess Publishing Company.
Campbell, L., Campbell, B., & Dickinson, D. (1992). *Teaching and learning through multiple intelligences.* New Horizon, WA.
Gardner, H. *Frames of Mind.*

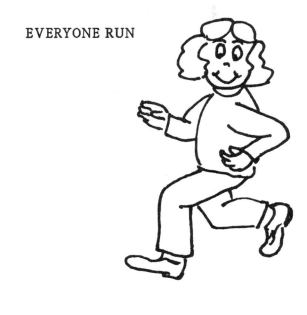

EVERYONE RUN

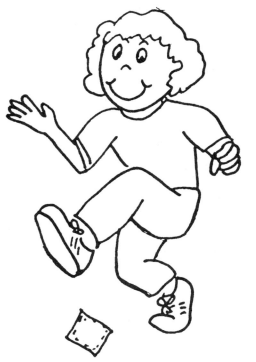

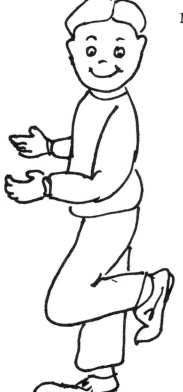

MARCH

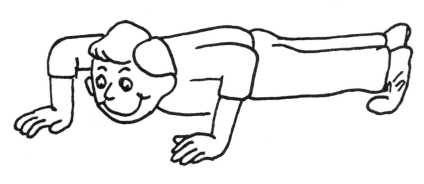

PUSH-UPS

SING A SONG IN THE KEY OF H FOR HEALTH†

Professional musicians seem to find it easy to motivate an audience to "sing a song." Take, for example, the following words from a popular Earth, Wind and Fire song:

> *When you feel down and out, sing a song.*
> *It'll make your day.*
> *You will learn to shout, in a song.*
> *It'll make you well.*
> *Sometimes it's hard to care, sing a song.*
> *It'll make your day.*
> *A smile is so hard to bear, sing a song.*

The lyrics are a melodic teacher, a helpful way of coping with the stressors of life, and the lessons are memorable. This musical example is not unique, however, because songs often promote learning in a direct (concrete), a second hand (vicarious), or an indirect (abstract) manner.

Although school health educators are not professional musicians, the inclusion of a variety of instructional strategies during health teaching should provide for concrete, vicarious, and abstract learning and promote the synthesis of health knowledge, attitudes and skills for living. Schools can "step to the beat of different drummers"—their own drummers—through creative orchestration. Both teachers and students can follow a step-by-step plan to design and implement health songs in the classroom.

Related Literature

It is essential for health educators to select teaching strategies which will lead to the attainment of health knowledge, skills, and attitudes. Health education and teacher education literature and research consistently support instructional variability, teacher enthusiasm, and creativity as being necessary for effective teaching. The utilization of music and lyrics during health instruction is a useful medium for motivating students to make personally satisfying, responsible health decisions. The inclusion of music and lyrics increases variability, enthusiasm, and creativity in teaching approaches. As Hochbaum (1978) states:

> *The purpose of teaching health is not to create knowledgeable children and adults. The purpose is to create healthy children and adults.*

Categorical curricula recently developed by many health related organizations—the American Automobile Association (1981), the American Cancer Society (1977 & 1979), the American Dental Health Association (1982), the American Heart Association (1982a, 1982b), and the American Lung Association (1983)—include many instructional strategies teachers can choose for use in the classroom. Several of these include musical songs to increase student motivation and participation.

Health education and teacher education literature substantiates the incorporation of innovative, creative teaching techniques such as musical songs during health instruction. Therefore, the authors encourage health instructors to incorporate musical songs relevant to health instruction and to consider "orchestrating" their own songs to teach health.

The "Song" and Its Use

The following song, "The Tracks of Time," was written for use in the American Cancer Society's *On The Right Track,* middle school health education curriculum (Smith, 1984). It provides an example of how to write, chord, and use a musical song in health instruction. Also, one should note how adaptable the song can be for almost any health subject matter chosen for instruction.

---

†*By Dennis W. Smith, Health Educator with the Columbus Partnership for Adolescent Health at Children's Hospital, Columbus, OH, and Brenda Smith, Assistant Professor of Health Education, University of Toledo, Toledo, OH. This article was previously published in Health Education, August/September 1986, 17(4), 42-43.*

The Tracks of Time

C*
Moving on down the tracks of time
      E   F
Oh I feel so good and i look so fine
      C   G C
And it's right, all right.
C
I'm an engineer, I'm a son-of-a-gun
         E   F
And I'm on the track and I'm making a
good run
        C   G C
And it's right, all right
        G

Chorus:

    Switchman, switchman on the
    line
    C
    You tell me now which track is
    mine.
    G
    You shift the rail so I can see
    C   G   C
    the life that I want mine to be.

C
The track is curved in front of me
      E   F
Oh I need a friend right by my seat
        C G C
To make it right, all right.

Chorus
C
Moving on down the tracks of time
      E   F
Oh I feel so good and I look so fine
       C G C
And it's right, all right.
C
Life's trip is long and wide
      E   F
Oh I've got my guide to help me decide
      C G C
So it's right, all right.

*This letter represents the appropriate
chord for musical accompaniment.

Teaching Suggestions for "The Tracks of Time"

1. Play the tape, "The Tracks of Time" (Smith, 1984) on a regular basis. Encourage the students to sing the chorus and the last line of each verse (It's right, all right).

2. Bring in your own guitar and play/sing your own version of "The Tracks of Time" with your class. (The song was recorded in the key of D, capo up two frets, in the key of C).

3. Ask the following questions: What are the tracks of time? (Each person's life.) How are we engineers of our own trains? (Internal locus of control.) Is any health choice all right? (Responsible decision-making.) Who is the switchman? (A health educated individual.) What are some of the curves we face on the tracks of time? (Setbacks, milestones, challenges to our health choices, diseases, peer influences.) Who is the guide right by our side? (Switchman, personal value system.)

4. Encourage your students to illustrate their own personal "Tracks of Time."

5. Encourage your students to role play the different themes shared in the song.

6. Relate the "Tracks of Time" to the entire American Cancer Society's curriculum for health education, *On The Right Track* (Smith, 1984).

Original Songs—A Four Step Process

Step I: Think about the health unit or subject matter. Write key words such as friends, decisions, love sharing, vitamins, pollution, that you might want to include in your song. Include suggestions from your students if possible. Keep in mind that this is a lesson planning phase as far as appropriate content, grade level, and curriculum considerations are concerned. Songs are appropriate at any age. As a general rule, however, the younger the audience, the more simple the composition should be. Also, older students may be a bit shy to participate. With a bit of encouragement, they will probably enjoy the experience.

Step II: Create a tune. Hum, kazoo, or strum a sequence of melodies that sound unique to you. A favorite method in Step II is to play compatible guitar chords and invent notes at random. This is relaxing and fun, but quite tricky to recreate. Pay attention to what is happening and let your ears guide you to a tune that you can replicate. "Pop" songs can lend ideas to this process. Variations of these songs can be used. However, credibility and satisfaction is gained from creating your own composition. Remember that not everyone can be a musician. Individual abilities may limit the development of a musical creation, but not the idea itself. Talented students can also help the teacher with musical limitations.

Step III: Combine Step I and Step II. Let your melody and words blend in poetic synergy by adding key words to rhythmic phrases such as:

Oh I've got my guide
to help me decide.
So it's right, all right.

Notice that key words can take different forms —decisions/decide—and attempt to rhyme the phrases, thus keeping continuity and meter.

Step IV: Instrumentation and recording. Instrumentation need not be elaborate. Guitars are popular choices. Also, bells, banjos, sticks, and even acappella accompaniment present pleasant combinations.

Recording the orchestration is an important consideration. Reel-to-reel tape recorders, small cassettes, and large portable cassette tape players are adequate recording devices.

The Musical Experience

Experiment with "creative orchestration" and discover possible untapped talents. The following suggestions lend further assistance in the use of music in the class:

Use quality audio equipment to play the music; make copies of the lyrics for the class; be receptive to other interpretations of the music from your students; be aware that misconceptions may be conveyed in your music; and, be aware that any teaching strategy can become ineffective if overused.

Songs produce a lasting effect on the listener. Many people find themselves remembering various melodies and lyrics from the past, discovering they are tapping their feet and singing words to songs that have not been heard for years. Many health educators and their students will discover that they have the ability to creatively write and orchestrate music relevant to health education. Although the resulting songs may not make the "Top 20," students and teachers will find their creative efforts memorable and rewarding. Students will be learning concretely, vicariously, and abstractly, promoting health concept formation and the development of healthy lifestyles. Also, musical methodology supports aspects of effective teaching behavior such as teacher variability and enthusiasm.

As the "conductor" of the health education experience, teaching methodology can take a variety of forms. When an "encore" event is desired in your class, "tune up" your talents, wave your wand, and sing a song. Your audience will applaud for life!

References

American Automobile Association. (1981). *Starting early: Alcohol and safety education, K-6 and Al-Co-Hol, 7 & 8.* Traffic Safety Department, Falls Church, VA.

American Cancer Society, Inc. (1979). *An early start to good health, K-3.* (Contact Regional Cancer Society.)

American Cancer Society, Inc. (1979). *Health networks, 4-6.* (Contact Regional Cancer Society).

American Dental Association. (1982). *Learning about your oral health, Preschool-12.* Chicago, IL.

American Heart Association. (1982). *Putting your heart into the curriculum, K-12.* Dallas, TX.

American Heart Association Subcommittee on Health Education of the Young. (1982). We've put our heart into the curriculum. *Health Education,* January-February, 20-21.

American Lung Association. (1983). *Lungs are for Life.* (Contact Regional Lung Association.)

Health Activities Program. Northbrook, IL: Hubbard, P.O. Box 104.

Hochbaum, Godfrey H. (1978). Some select aspects of school health education. *Health Education,* March-April, 31-33.

Smith Dennis W. (1984). "The tracks of time." *On the Right Track.* American Cancer Society Health Education Curriculum, Columbus, OH.

THE HEALTH REPORTER POOL†

Students, who are often viewed as "receptacles" in which to deposit health-related information, should be more actively involved in the learning process. A primary problem with mass-produced teacher guides and curriculum manuals in health education is that they tend to focus more on subject matter than on student participation. The field of health education, however, presents many opportunities to actively involve the student in the learning process. The goals of health education differ from other subjects, such as mathematics, geography, or history, where knowledge is factual and cumulative. In health education, knowledge should be combined with efforts to influence positive health attitudes, effective decision-making skills, and promotion of positive health behavior.

The Health Reporter Pool is an activity that can combine a variety of student-centered activities into a single lesson format. The central idea of the Health Reporter Pool activity is that a student is selected to role play a particular health-related "character." The choices for characters are limitless, for example, a bacterium, a carbohydrate, a drug abuser, a positive self-esteem, a good decision, or the human immunodeficiency virus (HIV). Based on class size, a number of other students are selected to be reporters "assigned" to cover a press conference, in the presence of the class, with each health-related character.

Several days prior to the press conference, the character and the reporters conduct research to discover facts and other health-related issues pertaining to the character. Reporters must formulate relevant questions such as: "What is it like to be a bacterium?"; "What good do you do anyone?"; or "If you are supposed to help humans, why do you constantly have to be controlled?" The teacher can limit or expand the types and number of questions based on availability of time and resources.

An exchange between the reporters (R) and the character (C) might go as follows:

R1:   "So tell me, what makes you, a bacterium, so important?"
C: "Well, I am very important in helping the body conduct a variety of functions."
R2:   "Would you be so kind as to elaborate on two or three of these functions?"
C: "First of all, I assist the intestinal tract in the digestion of food. In addition, I can help ward off certain infectious organisms."
R3:   "Please describe your relationship with antibiotic drugs."
C: "As you may be aware, I've never really enjoyed being around antibiotics, and I'll tell you why. . . ."

The Health Reporter Pool can be used with a variety of grade levels (7-12) and diverse ability groups. In addition, this activity is structured with maximum flexibility to allow the teacher to fit it into specific time frames and availability of resources. For example, the activity can be used as a 10-minute introduction to a new unit or as an entire class session on a particular topic. Also, the teacher can design questions for the participants to research or rely on the students to generate their own set of questions and responses. Most importantly, no special materials are needed for this activity, although students should be encouraged to use appropriate props to represent their specific character.

Advantages of using the Health Reporter Pool are numerous. First, it actively involves students in the learning process. Health class then becomes "something to do," rather than "something to attend." Students become involved in researching a particular subject for something besides a research paper or other written report. Second, topics that many students might consider boring (e.g., nutrition, infectious disease, personal health) can be made exciting and fun. In addition, controversial topics (e.g., AIDS, sexuality, substance abuse) can be approached from an impersonal perspective that could serve to reduce the inherent volatility of many of these issues. Third, the activity can be used with special populations. For example, classes comprised of a predominantly minority population can examine health care issues from the perspective of that particular group and even carry on the interview in a language other than English.

---

†By David Wiley, teacher at Southwest Texas State University, San Marcos, TX. This article was previously published in the Journal of Health Education, November/December 1992, 23(7), 433-434.

Fourth, the Health Reporter Pool can be used to integrate health with other content areas. As an example, the problem of AIDS can be examined from a sociological perspective, with the health educator and sociology teacher using the Pool to serve as an introductory activity in a coordinated effort to provide a focus on the topic. Thus the activity provides a medium to spread the health education curriculum across related content areas within a school. Fifth, students must learn beyond rote memorization and advance to higher level thinking and interaction skills. With the Health Reporter Pool, students learn to answer a range of questions focused on advancing discussion beyond basic facts.

Finally, students have the opportunity to develop public speaking skills. For many students, speaking before a group is a very uncomfortable experience. By structuring the activity carefully, the teacher can provide students with the opportunity to practice speaking in a controlled environment. For those students who speak comfortably in front of a group, the Pool provides an opportunity to ad lib and have fun creating an interesting interview.

The Health Reporter Pool idea has the potential for use in a variety of ways. Teachers have the discretion to use the activity in a strictly controlled manner or to allow students to construct their own interviewing activity. As this activity is used throughout the school year, the more comfortable and creative students can become in its use.

Its most important characteristic is that it directly involves students in the process of learning. The Health Reporter Pool provides teachers with a creative and challenging activity in which students may develop new skills while refining skills that already exist.

LIVING HISTORY . . .
THE GALLERY OF HEALTH CHAMPIONS†

The contributions of individuals towards the well-being of people from ancient to modern times is an important facet of health education at the intermediate grade level. In order to foster knowledge and appreciation of health's heritage, students need to recognize those men and women who, having fought and vanquished ignorance, prejudice and frustration in their battle against ill-health and disease, stand as health's champions.

Making health's history come alive for students is the unique dramatic presentation, "The Gallery of Health Champions." This activity not only brings the contributions of these health heroes and heroines to the attention of the students but also fosters student participation and learnings. Health educators have long known the advantages of dramatic presentations (mime, role-playing, skits, and plays) for making health concepts more readily understandable for their pupils. "Children are more likely to remember facts when they are portraying them" (Cornacchia, Olsen & Nickerson, 1989, 283).

The Gallery varies from the stage format generally followed from fourth through the sixth grades. Firstly, it is a multi-disciplinary (art, social studies and language arts), group-centered project that is designed, researched, written, produced, and performed by students involving cooperative learning, expository (historical inquiry and reporting), and expressive (play design, plot and dialogue) writing and the constructive arts (sets, costumes and properties).

Secondly, the production employs the theatre-in-the-round model. Individual sets representing a specific health champion are placed on and adjacent to the walls with the performers, frozen in statue-like positions, providing a three-dimensional form to each setting. This complements the Gallery theme in which spectators walk around to view the in-place pictures and sculptures. Because

†By Eleanor B. English, Ed.D., St. Bonaventure University, St. Bonaventure, NY.

of this design, the play does not require an auditorium/stage arrangement and works best in a classroom, all-purpose room or gymnasium. This environ allows the audience, depending on its number, to either walk around with the museum curator to each set or to turn, while sitting on the floor, to visually follow the curator's tour to the individual champion's set. Each set remains a still-picture until introduced by the curator. The performers come to life and present the researched historical data, that has been written with dialogue in the playlet form.

The third unique facet of The Gallery is its design, which allows the audience to become part of the production, either in asking questions directly to the performers (who may leave the set to roam through the audience while responding to or eliciting questions) or by involving themselves singularly or in groups with the action of the "picture." The latter may take place in several creative ways, e.g., a member of the audience might be asked to come to the set to view into a microscope and report the findings or someone might be asked to come forth and have a "war wound" bandaged by Florence Nightingale, etc. Not knowing who will be invited to perform or what actions will be called upon further heightens the audience's interest in the play and fosters a personalization and empathy with the champions. Once this process has occurred, learnings are enhanced (Ceprano & English, 1990, 67).

A schema, accompanied by a model playlet and samples of Gallery sets, is given as a guide for teachers/students for a successful presentation before other classes and parents or as a part of a health fair.

The Gallery of Health Champions: Schema

I. Introductory Phase (Teacher)
    A. Information Giving
        1. Introduces health's history and the individuals who played a significant role; notes the theme of health champions including a few people with their personal background within the historical context and their specific contributions to health.
        2. Details the sources of information available, e.g., encyclopedias, non-fiction and fiction tradebooks, medical history books appropriate for the grade level such as *Famous Men of Medicine* (Chandler et al., 1950).
        3. Compiles and presents a list of health champions which includes both well-known and little-known (e.g., Vesalius, Mary Walker, etc.) men and women throughout a broad time span. A sample list might include the following: Hippocrates; Andreas Vesalius; William Hervey, Edward Jenner; Florence Nightingale; Joseph Lister; Catharine Beecher; Elizabeth Blackwell; Sally Tompkins; Clara Barton; William Rontgen; Marie Curie; Frederick Banting; and Alexander Fleming.
    B. Task Presentation
        1. Defines the task; sets groups (no more than five pupils in each); appoints leaders; and sets group responsibilities and time limits.
        2. Directs a reading and talk-through of the sample playlet which acquaints students with the overall play format.
        3. Guides and assists the groups through the subsequent Phases.

II. Preparation Phase (Students)
    A. Audition for role of Curator; class selects the best performer.
    B. Each group selects the champion they wish to dramatize. The number of champions portrayed depends on class size.
    C. Activate the inquiry process (social studies):
        1. Brainstorm questions concerning the champion (birth, death, family, education, research, personal motivation, accomplishments) and historical period (language, clothing, transportation, prevalent diseases, medical treatment available); list most relevant questions; and search and collect data to determine answers.
        2. Analyze the gathered data; choose pertinent data for inclusion in the playlet.
    D. Compose the playlet utilizing expository writing in an expressive manner (Language Arts).
    E. Audition for roles in the playlet; performers are selected by the group's leader who acts in the capacity of director/producer.

III. Production Phase (Students)
  A. Sets/Costumes/Properties (note photographs)
    1. Based on the research, all three of the above should best represent the historical period in the most simple manner.
    2. Each historical vignette is located on an individual set designed as a three-sided (5x4x5) picture frame of black construction paper attached to the wall. Newsprint paper or cloth is adhered to the base of the wall and extended three feet outward on the floor. Appropriate drawings or properties may be placed within the picture frame. A sign denoting the champion's name and accomplishment stands on a tripod to the side of each set. Regular classroom lighting may be used. If available, a portable spotlight placed in the center of the room would be most effective.
    3. Collect and/or make simple costumes. Pictures of the period help in matching the dress of the champion.

IV. The Presentation Phase (Students)

V. The Post-Play Evaluation (Teacher and Students)

The Gallery of Health Champions
(A Sample Playlet)
(Performers in the picture frames are in place;
Curator enters room)

<u>CURATOR</u>: Welcome ladies and gentlemen, boys and girls, to this special place where history comes alive . . . the Gallery of Health Champions! You have the opportunity not only to see these people who battled against the forces of ill-health and disease to make life more healthy for people of all ages but to also ask questions of them concerning their contributions. You may even be called upon to perform some type of actions connected with their work in health. Come along with me now as we tour the Gallery of Health Champions. (Walks to Catherine Beecher's set.) Here is the picture of our first champion, Catherine Beecher, who noted the importance of exercise for good health.

<u>BEECHER</u>: Hello, my name is Catherine Beecher. When I opened my school for young girls in 1822, not only was education for females considered unnecessary, but physical exercise and activity were also discouraged by society. The fashions of this time, with their tight wasp-waists and enormous hoop skirts made any strenuous physical activity almost an impossibility. As a result of this, I found that much too often my students appeared to be pale, listless, too easily fatigued after too little work, and often susceptible to communicable diseases. I strongly believed that daily physical exercise while wearing loose, free-flowing clothing would promote good health. But what type of exercises would be most beneficial for my young women? I investigated

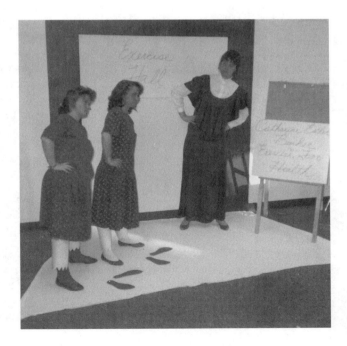

CATHERINE E. BEECHER
Exercise for Health

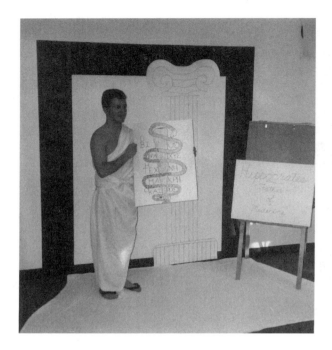

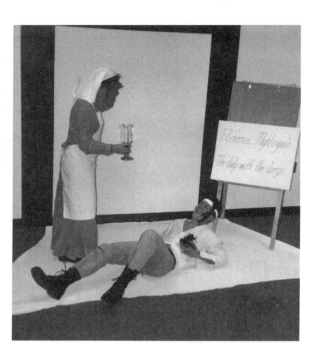

HIPPOCRATES

Father of Medicine

FLORENCE NIGHTINGALE

The Lady With the Lamp

the German System of Gymnastics and found all that vaulting over stuffed horses to be too strenuous and dangerous for females. I decided to design my own system of calisthenics, originally for females, but now modified for use in schools and with families at home. Watch carefully as my students demonstrate a few here in the Seminary Exercise Hall. See the footprints placed on the floor? Those are there for students to stand on so as to be given room to move. Sometimes we perform these movements to music. Ready girls? Begin. (Two students follow Beecher's direction and do three forms of her exercises; on completion, Beecher turns and addresses the audience.) Now, I want the audience to stand, watch, and do a few of my exercises with me. Ready, begin! (She leads audience in a few exercises.) Remember to always exercise your way to good health. (Returns to frozen position within the picture frame; the Curator enters.)

CURATOR: Through her books and articles, Catherine Beecher remained a strong champion of exercise for good health. (Turns to set #2.) Now turn your attention to the next picture. Within this frame you will see the inventor of the stethoscope, Theophile Laennec. He will explain how he came to design this very important health instrument.

References

Ceprano, M., & English, E. B. (1990, Winter). Fact and fiction: Personalizing social studies through the textbook tradebook connection. *Reading Horizons.*

Cornachhia, H. J., Olsen, L. K., & Nickerson, C. (1989). *Health in elementary schools* , 7th ed. St. Louis: Times Mirror/Mosby College Publishing.

Chandler, C. A. (1950). *Famous men of medicine.* New York: Dodd, Mead and Company.

ENVIRONMENTAL HEALTH AND MATHEMATICS: MAKING CONNECTIONS IN THE CLASSROOM†

During the early 1990s the nation's headlines repeatedly contained news of oil spills, water and air pollution, deforestation, and solid waste disposal problems. These and other environmental health concerns are receiving increased emphasis in school curricula and in school recycling and conservation projects (Texley, 1990). Another emphasis that has accompanied entry into the new decade is the call for reform in school mathematics, as evidenced in the new *Curriculum and Evaluation Standards for School Mathematics* by the National Council of Teachers of Mathematics (1989). These two movements present teachers with a timely opportunity to interrelate the two subjects in innovative ways for their K-8 students.

The purpose of this article is to suggest some introductory activities for making connections between environmental health and mathematics. In a sense, the two subjects can serve in complementary roles. The context of environmental health can serve to motivate students to develop mathematical concepts and skills. The formulas and processes of mathematics can serve to model and quantify many phenomena associated with environmental health. It is hoped that as students make connections between the two subjects, their knowledge and understanding of each will be enhanced.

Activity 1

This activity demonstrates that a substantial amount of water can be saved if K-8 students will turn off the water while brushing their teeth, rather than allowing the water to run continuously. Begin the activity by asking each student to brush his/her teeth three times, using water to wet the brush and rinse only. Catch the water used during each brushing in a one-quart container, such as a standard mayonnaise jar. Estimate the amount used each time to the nearest one-fourth of a quart and record the data in a table. An example is given in Figure 1. The column labeled "Average" in Figure 1 gives the average amount of water used per brushing.

Figure 1	**TURNING WATER ON AND OFF**			
Brushing	#1	#2	#3	Average
Amount of Water	1/2 qt.	3/4 qt.	1/4 qt.	1/2 qt.

Repeat the process for three more brushings, this time allowing the water to run continuously. Again, record the data in a table. An example is given in Figure 2.

Figure 2	**WATER RUNNING CONTINUOUSLY**			
Brushing	#1	#2	#3	Average
Amount of Water	4 1/2 qts.	4 qts.	3 1/2 qts.	4 qts.

The results of the two examples reveal that a student who turns the water off while brushing uses an average of 1/2 quart per brushing; the same student letting the water run continuously uses an average of 4 quarts, or one gallon, per brushing. The students will be surprised that they use <u>eight</u> times as much water if the water is allowed to run continuously!

---

†*By Charlene K. Stewart and James F. Strickland, Jr., Georgia Southern University, Statesboro, GA.*

Students not yet familiar with fractional number computations can visually compare the amounts of water used in the two processes. Again, the conclusion can be drawn that much more water is used by letting it run continuously. Teachers can extend this activity by asking questions such as: "How much water could you save, as an individual, in one year by using the on-and-off technique?" and "How much water could our class save in one week?"

Activity 2

The second activity focuses on recycling aluminum cans. Have students bring empty soft drink cans to school for a hands-on lesson. Lead students to understand that a soft drink can is a concrete model of a cylinder, with circular-shaped bases and a rectangular-shaped lateral surface. Provide students with rulers to measure the diameter (d) of a base and the height (h) of the can. Students may now compute the volume of the can using the formula $V = \pi r^2 h$, where $r = d/2$.

The formula will seem very abstract and of little relevance to some students. Teachers can add meaning to the concept of volume by asking students to think of it as the amount of soft drink that can be packaged again and again when new cans are made from recycled aluminum. Students will enjoy conjecturing how many liters or gallons of their favorite soft drink might be consumed while an important natural resource is being conserved.

Recycling aluminum cans has become a popular money-making project in some schools. Profits are often used to purchase computers, calculators, and other instructional aids. Many mathematical skills in estimating and computing can be further developed in a class or school recycling project.

Activity 3

The third activity concerns noise pollution. High volume stereo systems provide one source of noise pollution to which most middle school students are exposed. The detrimental effect of listening to loud music for a short time period is immediate but not lasting. The detrimental effect becomes lasting when one listens to high volumes frequently and for long periods of time. An impressive activity demonstrating the potential danger of such practices can be safely experienced by K-8 students. *Step 1*—(a) Place a loud-clicking timer at a prescribed point. (b) Allow the students to move away from the clicking timer to the point when they can no longer hear it. (c) Mark, measure, and record the individual students' "hearing distances." *Step 2*—(a) Place a very loud source of music (students' favorite rock number) near the students for several minutes. (b) Immediately repeat Step 1. (c) Compare findings in Step 2 with those of Step 1.

Several additional studies can be completed by manipulating noise volume and length of listening time and by comparing students' "listening distances" along with their daily music listening habits.

Using the activities described in this article can benefit your students in a variety of ways. They will become better informed about environmental health issues. They will identify specific actions they can take to conserve natural resources and improve the environment. They will apply mathematical concepts and skills in meaningful ways. And, they will see connections between environmental health and mathematics, two disciplines which heretofore may have seemed unrelated.

References

National Council of Teachers of Mathematics. (1989). *Curriculum and Evaluation Standards for School Mathematics.* Reston, VA: NCTM.

Textley, Juliana. (1990, February). Practice what you teach. *The Science Teacher, 57,* 39-41.

TEACHING THE DIGESTIVE SYSTEM IN ELEMENTARY PHYSICAL EDUCATION†

Currently, the holistic approach, or integrating physical education with academic subjects, is being stressed as a part of a good physical education curriculum. In January 1987, an article was published in *Journal of Physical Education, Recreation, and Dance* explaining and demonstrating an active, inexpensive way to teach the circulatory system (Kern, 1987). Perhaps even before 1987, but definitely since then, other circulation models have been constructed. Although the circulatory system is one of the main body systems one associates with physical activity, the digestive system can also be learned through activity. As physical educators profess, "we learn best by doing."

Following Kern's model where the students are the blood in the circulatory system, in the digestive system, each student is a piece of food. In this inexpensive model, the only equipment needed is: mats on which the students do sit-ups or push-ups representing chewing, signs (preferably laminated) to identify the major structures of the digestive system, chairs on which the signs are taped and to separate the "good food" from the waste," and cones—small ones to keep students safely in the appropriate areas and large ones to help them know when to leave the system to return to become a new piece of food.

The main concepts taught are: (1) the food is chewed in the mouth; (2) the food then passes through the esophagus to the stomach to the small intestine; (3) the food the body absorbs into the blood "gets in" at the small intestine; (4) the waste not absorbed in the blood passes through to the large intestine, rectum, and out through the anus (or simply "out" after the large intestine).

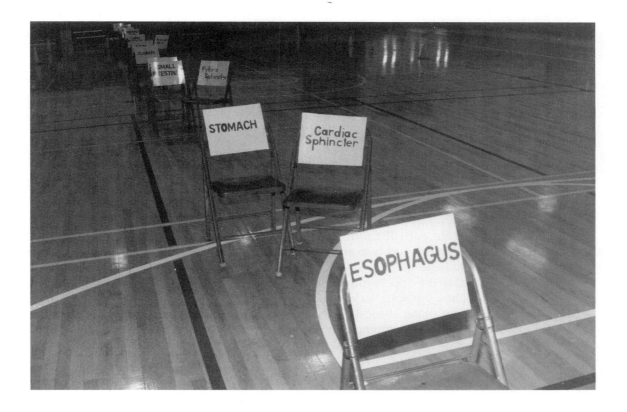

†*By Sue Moen, Ph.D., Dallas Baptist University Lab School, Dallas, TX.*

Before becoming a new piece of food to be chewed up (5-10 sit-ups or push-ups), the children decide whether they want to be the "good stuff" (to be absorbed at the small intestine) running down the <u>right</u> side of the chairs or the "bad stuff" running down the <u>left</u> side of the chairs (and "out"). This prevents children from crossing between chairs and helps avoid safety problems.

Our kindergartners through second graders run through the system as previously discussed. They make sure they go <u>around</u> the cones by the mouth, because they know food cannot be taken in through the cheek!

For the older elementary children, additional signs are placed on chairs for the parts of the small intestine: the duodenum, jejunum, and ileum. Since most absorption takes place at the duodenum and jejunum, the cones marking the area through which they will leave are directly across from one of those signs. Additional signs can be used, too, for the four areas of the large intestine (colon): ascending colon, transverse colon, descending colon, and sigmoid colon.

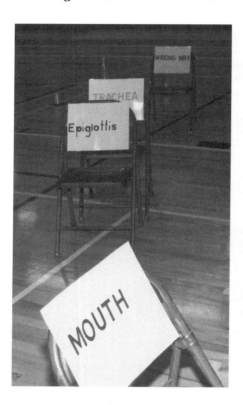
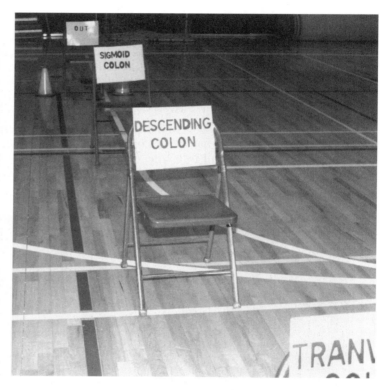

Later, other concepts are added: children of all ages find it fun to "throw up"; after "being chewed," they run to the stomach and turn and run right back out through the mouth. The concept of reverse peristalsis is taught here.

Older children later have the opportunity to learn about choking by taking an incorrect path, past the epiglottis into the trachea, but then back to the mouth and onto the correct path (or they can start over immediately as a new piece of food).The older children, too, can add jumping jacks in the esophagus to represent peristalsis, jumping jacks in the stomach for the muscle action on chyme, and running in place just before entering the small intestine while they wait for the pyloric sphincter to open. Signs are used for the cardiac sphincter and ileocecal valve as well as for the pyloric sphincter. Also, whether signs for the rectum and anus are used or simply the sign "out," the children can run in place while waiting for the rectal muscles to relax and the anus to open.

If enough space is available, the digestive and circulatory systems could be combined by having the children who get "absorbed" leave the digestive system and enter the circulatory system. In this way, the children would learn about how the systems are "integrated." Possibly, the respiratory system could also be added.

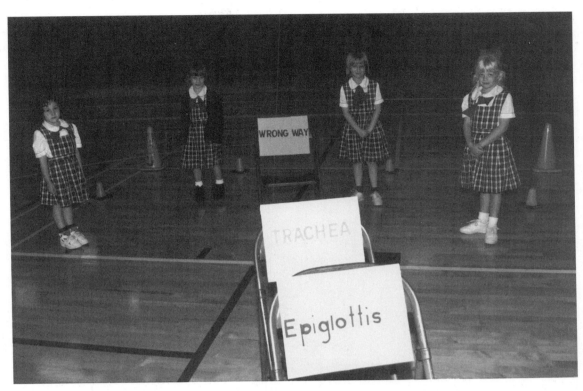

For a cooldown to this lesson, the children walk through the system a few times and then stretch. In the review, children are asked questions about the system. After only two or three days (non-consecutive), I have found that most kindergartners can describe the digestive path as "mouth, esophagus, stomach, small intestine, large intestine, and out," and they know that the "good stuff" is absorbed into the blood at the small intestine.

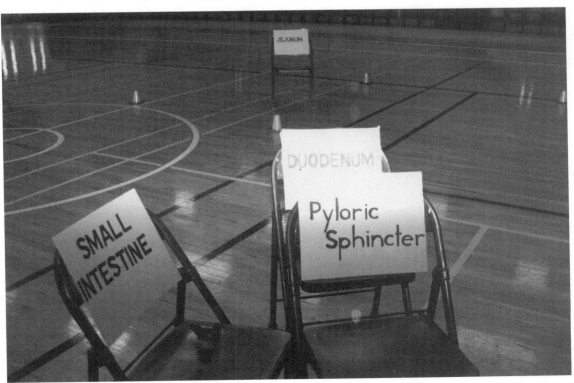

In this lesson, the children have a maximum amount of participation time including a warm-up (walking and then jogging slowly through the system as a review), at least 10-15 minutes of time during which their heartrates are consistently raised, several different sets of sit-ups and push-ups, a cooldown (same as the warm-up), and static stretching at the end of class. Most of the children find this an enjoyable lesson and will let me know when they are <u>reviewing</u> the digestive system in their classroom, after having already learned it in the gym!

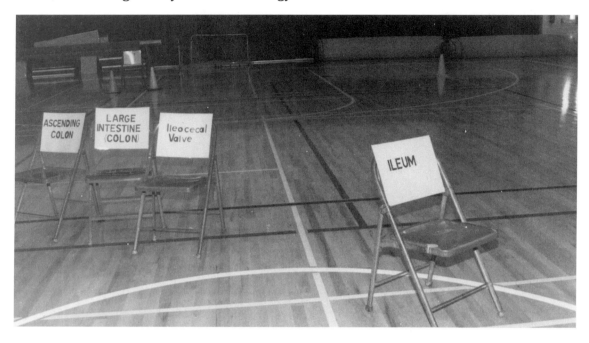

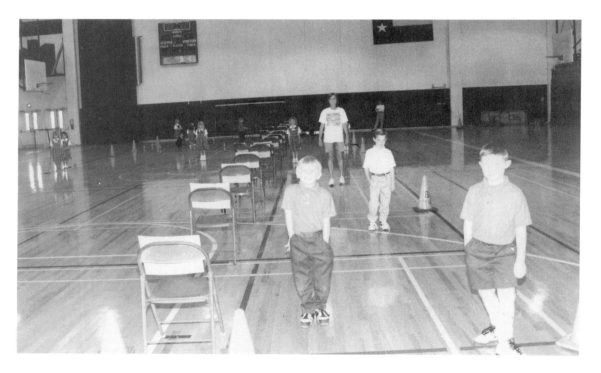

Reference: Kern, Kathleen, A. (1987, January). Teaching circulation in elementary P.E. classes. *Journal of Physical Education, Recreation, and Dance*, 62-63.

AN INTEGRATED APPROACH TO HUMAN GROWTH AND DEVELOPMENT†

Teachers face an ever-increasing schedule of required syllabi and topics competing for space in the shrinking school day. Interdisciplinary approaches to instruction have been developed to meet these challenges.

Why an integrated approach? Because learning, like health, occurs all the time, not just in neat 45-minute segments. Integration is a microcosm of life, offering flexibility, meaningful correlation, and inter-subject reinforcement. For maximum impact, team planning, implementation and evaluation should be initiated.

Health education does not exist in a vacuum; by utilizing an integrated approach, educators can help students to make connections between similar concepts presented in different ways. This maximizes learning, retention and application. Students see educators cooperating and communicating, visible role models in real life.

A single lesson may be piloted, or an integrated unit, theme-based activity or day can be created. In a similar manner, selected skills can be taught and reinforced through several subject areas. Teachers can create unifying themes for a semester or year.

There are many ways to meet subject objectives through integrated approaches. For shared/mutual integrated applications, syllabi, curricula and collateral materials need to be reviewed to identify mutual goals and objectives. Many of these will be very similar; many will be complementary. These goals and objectives can then be achieved through a planned interdisciplinary approach.

Activities can be planned around a theme, such as "family membership" or "rules and responsibilities" which can be developed in many subject areas. If themes are clearly articulated and reinforced across the curricula, students will make appropriate learning connections, assisted by educators in several disciplines.

The following activities can be used as part of a unit on human growth and development in the elementary or middle school.

Ages and Stages: An Exploration

For interdisciplinary curriculum planning, this lesson encompasses mathematics, language arts, social studies, and art, in addition to health. This activity is particularly suitable for special education students.

There are two instructional objectives: the student will (1) identify classifications as gender and age, (2) describe and compare a range of roles and capabilities for people of all ages and genders.

Prior to this activity, collect a stack of magazines or catalogues containing numerous pictures of people of all ages. Also needed: posterboard or construction paper, staples or glue.

Step 1: Ask students to look through magazines and catalogues and cut out pictures of infants, boys, girls, men and women of all ages. Mount pictures one at a time on posterboard or chart paper. As they finish, classify and divide pictures into these approximate categories: infant, toddler, child, pre-teenager, teenager, young adult, adult, senior citizen. Look for a distribution of males and females in each category, if possible. Do not discuss these categories with the class as you classify; let them come to their own conclusions as to ages—that's part of the fun!)

Step 2: Divide students into groups of 2 or 3 and give each group a selection of 4-5 different aged/gendered pictures to work with. With a 10-12 minute time limit, ask students to look at each picture, and decide:

(a) two activities that this person can definitely do;
(b) two activities that this person probably cannot do.

---

†*By Isabel Burk, M.S., CHES, Regional Drug Education Coordinator for Putnam/No. Westchester Board of Cooperative Educational Services, Yorktown, NY.*

Groups record their answers on the chart paper/poster. Then ask the groups, one at a time, to act out their "ages and stages" for each picture, for the class. (This will be a lot of fun and very revealing.)

Discuss their ideas and ask groups how they came to their answers. Explore the concept that age and gender do not rigidly define behaviors and skills. Ask: Do all toddlers learn to walk on their first birthday? Does every six-year-old learn to ride a two-wheeled bicycle on the same day? Do all elderly people use a cane to walk? Help students to see that abilities aren't strictly age- or gender-related.

Step 3: Within their groups, ask students to develop a list of abilities that relate to their age group. Then ask them to develop a second list, a "wish list" of activities that they want to be able to do soon. (This might include driving, going to the movies without an adult, etc.) Collate the most common ideas into class lists and discuss similarities. This provides peer support and a public forum for students to discuss their future goals. Define "maturity," "responsibility" and "ability" and discuss their interrelationship.

How Long Do We Live?

Students in grades 3-6 are taking increasing responsibility for their health-related behaviors. To raise awareness of the long-term effects of their behaviors, this series of activities will produce both cognitive and affective results.

For interdisciplinary curriculum planning, this lesson encompasses mathematics, language arts and social studies in addition to health. This activity is also suitable for special education students. Several *World Almanacs* or similar reference books would be very helpful.

There are two instructional objectives: students will be able to (1) identify and describe factors that influence life expectancy, and (2) identify and describe specific behaviors which will enhance their personal life expectancy.

Step 1: Define life expectancy: The number of years an "average" person born at a certain time can expect to live.

Step 2: Give students the basic life expectancy numbers from Figure 1 (or ask students to research these figures).

Step 3: Have students graph these life spans as a line graph and a bar graph.

Step 4: Students can use the graphs to determine the change in life expectancy in the past two centuries. In small groups or as a class, discuss what factors may have influenced longevity. (Include technological factors such as modern medical science, improved transportation, improved access to medical care, literacy, diet, agricultural techniques, sanitation improvements, occupations, economic status, living conditions.)

Now contrast these figures with life expectancies of people in other nations. Students can use the *World Almanac* to find this information. Add selected life expectancies to students' graphs; for instance, in 1981, the life expectancy of a child born in Nepal was 45 years; a child born in Ghana was expected to live 52 years; a child born in Ireland could expect to live to be 73. Research other countries and discuss the factors relating to their expected life span.

Figure 1

EXAMPLES OF LIFE EXPECTANCIES OF AMERICANS FROM 1800-1991

An American born in:	could expect to live to:
1800	47.3 years
1970	71.1 years
1980	73.2 years
1991	74.9 years

Step 5: In pairs or individually, have students contrast human life spans with average life spans of animals. Figure 2 presents some selected expectancies; ask students to research others. Graph this information as well. Students can also make a time line of life expectancy for animals and humans on the blackboard.

Step 6: Lead a class discussion on how students can contribute to longer life span. Ask students to list specific actions that can help them to live longer. (Examples: low fat diet, regular exercise, recognize and deal with stress, etc.)

Figure 2

SAMPLE LIFE EXPECTANCIES FOR SELECTED ANIMALS

Animal	Life expectancy
ape	45 years
cat	14 years
wolf	15 years
gerbil	3 years

Step 7: Challenge students to look ahead and predict what will the average life span be for infants born in 2100? Have students write a creative short story about the future of medicine, health, living conditions, etc. that may impact life span in the future.

What's Your Pulse?

For interdisciplinary curriculum planning, this lesson encompasses mathematics, science, social studies, in addition to health. This activity is particularly suitable for special education students. A stopwatch or sweep second hand clock is needed.

There are two instructional objectives: students will (1) demonstrate the ability to find and record pulse rate and (2) be able to differentiate average pulse rates for persons of many ages.

Step 1: Review the steps in taking pulse: index and middle finger pressed lightly against the "pulse point" on side of the throat or inside of wrist.

In class, have each student take his/her pulse for 20 seconds, then multiply by 3 to get the beats per minute. Repeat the process to check accuracy. Record the class's pulse rates as dots on a graph.

Then assign students to take a sampling of pulses from people of all ages: adults, younger students, older students. Use different colors to indicate these pulses on the chart.

Look at the dots and discuss patterns. The approximate pulse rates at rest for sample age groups are:

Figure 3

PULSE RATES FOR SELECTED AGE GROUPS

Age	Beats per minute
Newborn	130-150
1 year	100-130
6 years	90-110
11 years	70-100
Adult	80-90

Figure 4

SAMPLE ANIMAL PULSE RATES

Animal	Beats per minute
parakeet	600-800
mouse	300-500
cat	120-140
dog	70-120
lion	40-50
elephant	25-50

Make sure that students understand that variation is <u>normal</u>, Note that pulse rate is directly related to blood volume and size of the body.

Ask selected students to perform such activities as jumping jacks, jogging in place, etc., and then compare their pulse rates with the previous "at rest" rates. Discuss what other factors may cause pulse rates to rise (fear, surprise, extreme emotion, physical exertion, etc.)

Now compare with animal pulse rates. (See Table 4.)

Graph these data alongside the human pulse rate data and compare. What conclusions do the students come to?

An Integrated Approach to Substance Abuse Prevention

Alcohol, tobacco and other drug prevention issues must be addressed by elementary school teachers as a federally mandated component of school instruction. The issue is where to fit this in, and how to make it part of an overall course of instruction. Interdisciplinary approaches to instruction have been developed to meet these challenges.

Why an integrated approach? Because learning, like health, occurs all the time, not just in neat 45-minute segments. Integration is a microcosm of life, offering flexibility, meaningful correlation and inter-subject reinforcement. Effective substance abuse prevention cannot take place in a two or four week unit; it should be infused throughout the curriculum during the entire year for optimum value.

Substance abuse prevention does not exist in a vacuum; by utilizing an integrated approach, educators can help students to make connections between similar concepts presented in different ways. Team planning, implementation and evaluation are most effective in preparing an integrated approach. Not only will teamwork maximize learning, retention and application, but it provides positive role modeling of educators cooperating and communicating.

A single lesson may be piloted, or an integrated unit, theme-based activity or day can be created. In a similar manner, selected skills can be taught and reinforced through several subject areas. Teachers can create unifying themes for a semester or year.

There are many ways to meet subject objectives through integrated approaches. For shared/mutual integrated applications, syllabi, curricula and collateral materials need to be reviewed to identify mutual goals and objectives. Many of these will be very similar; many will be complementary. These goals and objectives can then be achieved through a planned interdisciplinary approach.

Activities can be planned around a theme, such as "red ribbon week" or "rules and responsibilities" which can be developed in many subject areas. If themes are clearly articulated and reinforced across the curricula, students will make (or can be taught to make) appropriate learning connections, assisted by educators in several disciplines.

The following activities can be utilized as part of the alcohol/tobacco an other drug prevention program in the elementary or middle school.

How Much Is Too Much?

For interdisciplinary curriculum planning, this lesson encompasses mathematics and language arts. This activity is particularly suitable for special education students.

There are four instructional objectives: The student will (1) observe and practice reading and implementing written directions (such as on a recipe or medication label); (2) be able to explain how too much of a substance can be unpleasant and undesirable; (3) describe a spectrum of body cues and their relation to good health.

Prior to the lesson, you will need to assemble these materials: water, sugar, lemons (or lemon juice), ice, spoons, measuring spoons, paper cups. Introduce the concept of "recipe" with students, if they are not familiar with this term. Explain that a recipe provides a standard method of preparing food that will yield standard, predictable results.

Now review a lemonade recipe with students, either on blackboard or overhead. (Most recipes call for 3 cups of cold water, juice of 4 lemons, and 1/2 cup of sugar.) Ask students to assist you in measuring and mixing the lemon juice and water.

Emphasize the importance of careful measuring. Do not measure or add sugar initially, but tell the class that they will add sugar to the lemonade a little at a time. Ask a volunteer to sip a small amount of lemonade without sugar, and describe it in terms of sweetness ("not sweet at all").

Measure out 1 cup of lemon/water mixture. Now ask a student to add 1/2 teaspoon of sugar to this, mix, taste a very small amount of it, and describe it in terms of sweetness ("not very sweet"). Have the student mix in 1/2 teaspoon of sugar, taste and describe ("a little bit sweet"). Repeat five more times until the student says the lemonade is "very sweet." At this point, ask him/her to add just 1/2 teaspoon more and describe the drink ("too sweet").

Repeat the experiment with another student. Then allow students to use the standard recipe to prepare lemonade, taste, and report out.

Ask students to remember how the lemonade changed to "too sweet" in the first experience. How can we avoid this? Use a recipe; the recipe will yield uniform lemonade that tastes good every time!

Explore student experiences with "too much." Have any students ever eaten too much candy? Drunk too much soda? Stayed out too long in the sun? How did they feel? Did they learn anything from these experiences? Is it possible to have too much of something, even something enjoyable, like sweets?

Discuss the concept of individual differences, in terms of quantity: sweetness, volume of music, night time sleep needs, etc., emphasizing that each person has a personal preference or tolerance level.

Now discuss body signals and their importance to overall health. Ask students what clues their bodies give them when they're hungry, thirsty, tired, etc. How do body signals help us know our limits and modify our behavior?

Finally, correlate the lemonade experiment to safe use of medication. Both over-the-counter and prescription medications list appropriate dosages for children and adults. These dosages have been tested by scientists and doctors to make sure that they work properly and won't be harmful. Each measure (pill, liquid, capsule, tablet) is carefully formulated the same way each time, from a "recipe" so that it will work the same way each time. Remind students of the overload of sugar and tell them that too much medication will not help, but could even make a person sick. It is important to read and follow label directions. Only a medical professional should change a medication dosage level.

The Visible Difference: Teaching About Dosage

For interdisciplinary curriculum planning, this lesson encompasses science, mathematics, and language arts. This activity is particularly suitable for special education students.

Before you begin, you will need to assemble: bright red food coloring or concentrated dye, measuring spoons, 8 clear containers of varying sizes from very small (1 oz. size) to very large (quart), box from children's liquid pain reliever.

Ask students to arrange the containers in size order and fill with water. Let water bubbles settle until you can see through clearly.

Have students carefully measure one teaspoon of coloring into each container and stir carefully. The class should be able to observe marked color differences. Ask volunteers to describe the color hues, or ask students to draw and color diagrams to match the color concentrations they observe. The smallest vessel will be highly concentrated; the largest will have very little color change.

Now correlate this to human body size. Select a student to read the label on the liquid pain reliever, and note that dosage is designated by body weight. Why? Ask students to draw conclusions about medicine dosage, using the results of this experiment. If appropriate, read the labels on a variety of over-the-counter medications to show the pattern of larger dosage for older people—really a substitution for asking for weight!

Discuss factors that impact medication's effects. For instance, larger people have more blood volume which dilutes medication (just like the experiment)! Food in the stomach may slow down the medication's absorption. An individual's metabolism, age and activity level may also influence medication effects.

Finally, remind students that alcohol is a drug. What would be the effect of an ounce of pure alcohol on a smaller body (such as a child) as compared to the effect on a larger body? Why? (Relate this to the color concentration experiment.) What other factors might influence the effect? Emphasize that alcoholic beverages affect all people, but smaller people generally feel the effects more quickly and intensely.

References

Fogarty, R. (1991). *The mindful school: How to integrate the curricula.* Palatine, IL: IRI/Skylight Publishing.

Fogarty, R., Perkins, D., & Barell, J. (1992). *The mindful school: How to teach for transfer.* Palatine, IL: IRI/Skylight Publishing.

Jacobs, H. H. (1990). *Interdisciplinary Curriculum: Design and Implementation.* Alexandria, VA: ASCD.

Kovalik, S. (1993). *Integrated Thematic Instruction: The Model.* AZ: Kovalik & Associates.

Lloyd-Kolkin, D., & Hunter, L. (1990). *The Comprehensive School Health Sourcebook.* Menlo Park, CA: Health & Education Communication Consultants.

New York State Education Department. (1986). *Health Education Syllabus Grades K-12.* Albany, NY: Bureau of Curriculum Development.

New York State Education Department. (1986). *Drug Education Curriculum Grades K-6.* Albany, NY: Bureau of Curriculum Development.

Center for Substance Abuse Prevention. (1989). *Prevention Plus II: Tools for Creating and Sustaining Drug-Free Communities.* Rockville, MD: U.S. Department of Health and Human Services National Clearinghouse for Alcohol and Drug Information.

SKILL ENHANCEMENT

THE "HOW" OF HEALTH EDUCATION: INTRODUCING SOCIAL SKILLS TO STUDENTS†

Teaching young people how to lead healthier lives can be exciting for both teachers and students. Giving students current and accurate information is the "what" of health education. Giving them a repertoire of social skills to use that information is the "how" of health education.

"How do I tell my friend I don't want to go with him to the party and still look cool?" "How do I settle an argument with my mother so that we both get what we want?" "How do I keep myself from talking back to my teacher?" These are the kinds of questions students need answered. Students face tough situations and they need to know how to get out of them.

One of the specific social skills many people of all ages can benefit from is one found in the *Skillwise*™ program, published by the Comprehensive Health Education Foundation, and in several health education curricula, *The Refusal Skill for Self-Control*™. These are the steps of the skill, each step followed by a phrase skill-users can say to themselves:

(1) Stop what you're doing (e.g., "Stop." "Wait a minute.").

(2) Name the trouble (That's . . .").

(3) State the consequences ("If I do that . . .").

(4) Think of something else to do, and move away from the situation ("Instead, why don't I . . .").

(5) Give yourself credit for staying in control (e.g., "I did a good job." "I stayed in control." "I stayed safe.").

This skill, like other social skills, is taught most effectively when teachers follow a method of instruction that comprises the following sequence:

(1) Introduce the skill.

(2) Model the skill.

(3) Facilitate practice.

(4) Provide opportunities for students to "transfer" the skill outside the classroom.

Let's concentrate on the first step, without which none of the others may be meaningful: How do you introduce the skill so that your students are motivated to learn it?

First, give them a reason to learn. Establish a context for learning the skill. Ask your students how "controlling yourself" applies to the health unit they're studying. Ask students to make a list of what they've done in the past to control themselves. Establish that they're already using some effective techniques. Have students discuss in small groups the difficulties in controlling themselves. Reach a consensus with students that it would be helpful to have a consistent technique to use.

Second make it real for students. Ask them to think of a time when they wanted to control themselves but didn't. Say that you're going to show them a way to help them do that.

Show them the steps of *The Refusal Skill for Self-Control*™. Point out key phrases they can use until they become more comfortable with the steps of the skill.

---

†*By Bob Patterson, Coordinator of* Skillwise® *and* Here's Looking at You, 2000® *at Comprehensive Health Education Foundation, Seattle, WA. This article was previously published in the Journal of Health Education, November/December 1993 Supplement, S-49.*

Ask students to write the sentence "Learning a new skill takes time" with the hand they normally don't write with. Compare their experiences with learning a new skill.

After you've introduced the skill, you can model it so that students "see" the skill themselves. Finally, you can ask students to identify situations in their lives in which they might use the skill.

Introducing *The Refusal Skill for Self-Control*™ isn't much different from introducing any other skill, or, for that matter, any other subject. The more you can convince students that they have a reason to learn something, and the more you can make it real for them, the more they're going to want to learn it.

And, after all, isn't that what *you* want?

TEACHING CHILDREN ABOUT STRESS THROUGH MOVEMENT†

Stress management for children is a concern for teachers and parents today. Movement can be used to explore the physical stress reaction and coping mechanisms. Five activities are described for students K-6 that identify sources of stress, explore how they might demonstrate a feeling of stress through physical movement, describe a balanced lifestyle and learn to believe in themselves more.

Teachers today are seeing stress among our nation's youth. Dr. Hans Seyle might define the stress as a divergent physical or emotional response to external factors in the students' life. Such things as headaches, stomach aches, mood swings, belligerent behavior and poor attention span might be indicative of stress in the child's life (Reed 1984). Educators today are looking for ways to help children cope with stress.

Using movement to define and discuss stress is a tool in the process of helping students cope. Using movement as therapy is not new. In the 1950s Marion Chace started using dance therapy on individuals hospitalized for mental disorders. Chace (1975) used movement activity to increase patients' active involvement with others, work on attention span, release nervous energy in an acceptable manner, and to communicate feelings nonverbally.

Debra Landforce (1990) said that the body never lies. One can learn much about internal feelings through observing and listening to the body. Berstein noted (1972) how much we ascribe feelings to body parts. For instance, we hear sayings such as "the eyes are windows of the soul," "teeth are biting sarcasm," "something can't be swallowed," or "he's a pain in the neck."

Levy (1988), a noted dance therapist, suggests that movement can identify and unify divergent forces within the person. This is certainly the goal of stress management for children.

The following movement activities are designed for students in the upper elementary age group but can be equally instructive and fun for teacher education groups. These activities can accommodate large or small groups of students. The lesson can be completed in a one-hour lesson and needs no special materials.

Activity 1—Defining Stress

Objective: Students will seek to recognize the presence of stress by observing individuals' body language when under stress.

Start with a discussion how do people look when they feel upset? Have students take turns describing a recent stressful situation for them. Have the group give him or her feedback on how the body changed or looked while talking about the stressful situation.

Have students take a partner. With the partner, take turns designing a visual human model of a person under stress. It may be a family member, friend or the student. Give examples of situations to

†*By Christine Wilson Ahmed, M.S., Assistant Professor, Department of H.P.E.R., Missouri Western State College, St. Joseph, MO.*

model: under the stress of a test, going to the dentist or fighting with a sibling. Is it easy to show stress physically? Where do we each feel stress in our bodies? Have students share before continuing to the next activity.

Activity 2—Sources of Stress

Objective: Students should be able to identify a current source of stress after this activity.

Ask students to think of what brings out those feelings of stress. Have students work with a same size partner this time. Students can hold onto a long stick or each other at the elbow or shoulder if this doesn't disrupt class. Start by either pushing or pulling for a count of five seconds. At any time individuals want to quit they can say "stop" to their partner. Ask them to tell what areas in their life that they feel that same sense of struggle. Does it seem like a good struggle or a bad one? Emphasize that they have the control to "quit" struggling at any time.

Activity 3—Acting Out Stress

Objective: Students may recognize a way that they cope with stress without thinking about it normally.

Ask students to think of situations when they feel stressed; focus on either the situation or the feelings of stress. What actions might express what they would like to do as a symbolic physical response to stress. Examples of actions might be pushing, retreating, hiding, withdrawing, showing heaviness, hyperactivity, or stamping, pushing, chopping, or punching. Have the students pick out five or more movements that express a response toward stress. Demonstrate them to the class with perhaps a verbal explanation of the movements if students feel ready to share. They can also share this with a partner if the group is large. There are many different ways of responding to stress. What are some good ways and some not so good?

Activity 4—Finding Balance

Objective: Students will identify people, activities, or situations that give them a sense of peace or balance.

Start the activity by talking about balance in life—what things make us feel good. With a partner again, have the students demonstrate three positions where they feel balanced against each other. Have the partners show the balances to the class. After the class looks at each one, have each person tell what helps them feel relaxed or good, balanced.

Activity 5—Stressors Are Challenges

Objective: This activity seeks to help students grow in the belief that they are capable of coping with a challenge.

Self-efficacy may begin by becoming involved rather than retreating from a challenge. We are going to use the action of either a side hug, arm around the shoulder or perhaps raising inside arms up high standing next to a partner to symbolize acceptance of a stressor as one of life's challenges. They might shout a refrain, I am a "SUPER Kid" (Serene, Unwound, Peaceful, Energized, and Ready-to-go) to end the activity on a positive note. As an instructor, give yourself a long, deep breath and a mental pat on the back. You're a SUPER Kid Too.

In conclusion, this activity provides students with an opportunity to learn about stress through movement activities. The lesson works well with the Health Education unit focusing on stress management. Children as well as adults become involved participants in the learning experience.

References

Berstein, P. L. (1972). *Theory and methods in dance-movement therapy.* Dubuque: Kendall/Hunt.
Chace, M. (1975). *Marian Chace: Her papers.* American Dance Therapy Association.
Coe, K. (1988). *Superkid assembly activities of Longridge school.* Rochester, NY. Paper presented at the American Alliance of Health, Physical Education, Recreation and Dance convention, Boston, MA.

Levy. F. (1988). *Dance movement therapy: A healing act.* Reston, VA: American Alliance of Health, Physical Education, Recreation, and Dance.

Landforce, D. (1990, August). Personal Interview. University of Oregon, Eugene, OR.

Reed, S. (1984). Stress, what makes kids vulnerable? *Instructor, 94,* 28-32.

Seyle, H. (1956). *The stress of life.* New York: McGraw-Hill.

JOURNAL WRITING; INTRODUCING A COPING TECHNIQUE IN STRESS MANAGEMENT COURSES†

Stress management classes are typically designed to introduce a host of relaxation techniques to accompany and compliment theoretical concepts of stress reduction from psychophysiology to strategies for stress reduction. Although coping techniques comprise a large component of stress management skills, it is often difficult to practice the complete effectiveness of these in the classroom without the immanent presence of personal stressors which all individuals can relate to equally. One effective coping strategy which can be taught as an in-class exercise is journal writing.

The Concept

The word *journal* comes from the root word "journee" meaning a day's travel or to journey or travel. Journals originally started as a means of guidance on long trips as a record or orientation for a safe return passage. From Columbus to Lewis and Clark to today's astronauts, journal writing has been and continues to be a proven means of communication for personal guidance on each individual's journey through life.

Current research suggests that not only is journal writing good for the soul, a type of catharsis to express the full range of emotions, it is proven to be good for the body as well. Studies in which individuals kept journals and wrote about their frustrations and painful experiences revealed that, over time, they had less physical ailments (headaches, cramps, etc.) suggesting a new bond in the link between the mind and the body (Pennebaker, 1988, 1989).

Journal writing is perhaps the most profound coping skill available to provide and enhance the skill of self-awareness, the essential coping tool needed to not only identify personal stressors, but to work on the resolution process of these as well. Journal writing initiates a communication of self-reflection, a necessary step in the resolution process. To initiate the journal writing process alone can be difficult. One way to enhance this process is with a few journal writing themes which serve as catalysts to promote the self-awareness and soul searching process. A class exercise in journal writing also lends credence to the concept of solitude and quality time for the purpose of self-reflection.

The following are two journal themes that have proven effective as a catalyst for increased self-awareness and self-reflection.

Journal Themes

There are several themes that can promote a sense of self-reflection and self-awareness. Journal themes should include a general concept with several supporting concepts which help the individual initiate the soul searching process. Themes should include a brief explanation regarding the major concept, its importance to the self-exploration process and several questions which serve as a catalyst for reflection. The following are two themes which have proven to be extremely successful in the attempt to promote reflections on self-awareness.

---

†By *Dr. Brian Luke Seaward, Assistant Professor, Department of Health and Fitness, The American University, Washington, DC.*

A Gift from the Sea: This theme, regarding reflections on personal strengths and weaknesses, is based upon the book *Gift from the Sea* by Anne Morrow Lindberg. To start this class assignment, a few preparations need to be made in advance. First, create a sea shell collection. Include approximately twice the number of shells as there are students to provide an abundance to choose from. Shells of varying size, shape, and color for students to select from add significantly to this experience. Additional shells can be borrowed or even purchased from novelty shops to balance out your collection. Second, if possible, locate a tape recording of ocean waves. The rhythmical sounds are very relaxing and promote the reflection process. Next, locate a copy of Lindberg's book, *Gift from the Sea* (1976) and select a couple of passages to be read at the completion of this exercise. Lastly, create a handout (or write on a blackboard) a series of thought-provoking questions related to this theme. Questions may include the following: *Describe the shell you selected, its size, shape, color, and any distinguishing features that stand out. What attracted you to this particular shell? Shells act as a form of protection and security. Humans, too, have shells, although invisible to the eye. What is your shell like? Does it over-protect or is it a growing shell? Shells can be strong or weak. What are your strengths and weaknesses? Sometimes strengths can become weaknesses, perfectionism, for example. Do any of your strengths have the tendency to become weaknesses? How do your strengths and weaknesses assist or confound your ability to deal with stress?*

At the start of the exercise, place the shells on a large beach towel. Ask each student to approach the towel and select a shell. Explain the concept of the assignment from the nature of journal writing to the specific concept of the sea shell as a metaphor of strengths and weaknesses. Allow 20-30 minutes for students to complete the assignment. When they begin to reflect and write, play the recording of the ocean waves to enhance the mood of the exercise. At the completion, allow students a few moments to finish remaining thoughts. As shells are returned, read a few selected passages from Lindberg's book. A short dialogue regarding this exercise may follow by asking students to describe their impressions of the journal theme and what it meant to them.

Vision Question: This theme regards the concept of rites of passage. It is based on the Native American custom of a retreat to nature; a three-day excursion of self-reflection and solitude. A vision quest is an intense probing of one's life purpose and contribution to mankind. It promotes an affirmation of centeredness and connectiveness to the Mother Earth. In the Native American custom, a vision quest marks a significant rite of passage into adulthood, or a major life transition. This concept is very adaptable to all societies. In contemporary American culture there are many rites of passage. While many are celebrated in ceremony, many are not, with the most difficult experienced alone. Rites of passage are thought to include three critical phases: *severance,* a separation from former ways of thoughts, behaviors, people, places, etc.; *threshold,* a quest, a search for vision or understanding; and *incorporation,* a return to community with knowledge from the vision. The concept of rites of passage become increasingly important in high school, during college, and throughout one's adult life.

To begin this assignment, some preparations will certainly enhance this experience. First, a tangible catalyst to promote self-exploration is helpful. A collection of tumble stones, either polished gems or common garden stones, will lend itself to the concept of groundedness (polished stones can also symbolize the concept that resolution of stressors smoothes the rough edges of our being). Second, because this theme is derived from the culture of southwest American Indians, Native American flute music lends an exponential quality to this experience as students begin the reflection and writing process (Nakai, 1987). Next, if possible, locate a reference regarding the concept of the vision quest to read a few selected passages at the completion of the assignment (Foster & Little, 1988). Finally, a handout or blackboard notes to highlight the concept and provide a few soul-searching questions related to this theme. Questions may include the following: *What significant events to date would you consider to be included in your own rites of passage and why? What rites of passage are you in the midst of currently? What dragons are you doing battle with right now? Regarding the concepts of severance, threshold, and incorporation, what life passage are you in now, what phase are you entering or emerging from? In a vision quest, a new name is received from the mother earth. A name can also be a positive affirmation statement, a unique phrase which boosts self-esteem and gives the ego a solid sense of positive identity. What phrase or positive affirmation statement can you suggest as a morale booster to give you a solid sense of positive identity?*

As students begin to reflect and write, play the recording of the Native American flute music. Allow 20-30 minutes for the journal writing session. At the end of the writing period, as students return the stones, select a few passages to read to bring closure to this theme. A short discussion may add final closure as individuals who wish to share their impressions of this journal theme comment on this concept.

Conclusions

There are many types of coping techniques to effectively deal with stress. Each coping technique must be initiated with an increased sense of self-awareness. Journal writing is perhaps the most well suited for this purpose. In-class journal writing exercises lend credence and opportunity to this coping style. Unlike other coping mechanisms which may not prove effective in the classroom setting for all students, journal writing initiates and maintains a strong sense of self-awareness. Because of the personal nature of these themes, and the conceptual balance of honesty of communication and privacy to promote honesty, these perhaps should not be collected, rather left inside the journal for review of the writer to enhance the learning experience.

References

Foster, S., & Little, M. (1988). *The book of the vision quest.* New York: Prentice Hall.

Lindberg, A. M. (1976). *Gift from the sea.* New York: Vantage Press.

Nakai, R. C. (1987). *Earth spirit.* Phoenix, AZ: Canyon Records Productions.

Pennebaker, J. W. (1988). Disclosure of traumas and immune function: Health implications for psychotherapy. *Journal of Consulting and Clinical Psychology, 56,* 239-245.

Pennebaker, J. W. (1989). Confession, inhibition, and disease. *Advances in Experimental Social Psychology, 22,* 211-244.

HIV/AIDS PREVENTION

PERSONAL IMPACT: MAKING A CURRICULUM MEANINGFUL TO STUDENTS†

How It Works

"Hey, you wanna trade?"

Chris studied the laminated cards in his hand. They were all the same, a graphic of a rose. He liked the cards, didn't really want to give up any of them. But his classmate Debbie was insistent.

"Come on, let's trade."

He nodded, not saying anything. He selected one of the roses and gave it to her. She gave him a card from her hand; it was a pitchfork. Not bad, thought Chris.

He switched three more times in the activity, though he had 10 opportunities altogether. Later, Mr. Thorn held up facsimiles of the cards everyone had.

"This card," said Mr. Thorn, holding up a graphic of a penguin, "is 'happiness.' How many people either have this card in their hands right now or had it pass through their hands?"

Several of Chris's classmates raised their hands, and they traced a ball of yarn from one to the other, based on who gave the penguin card to whom.

"And this card," said Mr. Thorn, holding up a graphic of a bee, "is chicken pox." The procedure was repeated: the raised hands, the yarn.

Mr. Thorn held up a card with a pitchfork on it. "All right," he said, "let's suppose that this card is the AIDS virus. How many people have had this card in their hands?"

Chris knew it was just a card, but he felt as if he had been kicked in the gut.

What It Does

This activity is called "The Invisible Thread." It's part of a middle school lesson illustrating some of the factors influencing the transmission and spread of the AIDS virus in an AIDS prevention curriculum called Get Real About AIDS™, published by Comprehensive Health Education Foundation. In this simulation, students realized the following:

The more times they switched cards, the more they risked getting a "bad" card.

Sometimes there was pressure to switch cards.

No one knew at the time of the switches who had the "AIDS" card, even the person who had it.

Even if someone gave away the "AIDS" card after having received it from someone, that person was still counted as having the card.

Students gain an understanding of HIV/AIDS, of the nature of epidemics, and of their own predispositions toward succumbing to peer pressure. How is this different from reading about HIV/AIDS, from

---

†By Neal Starkman, writer and developer at Comprehensive Health Education Foundation, Seattle, WA. This article was previously published in the Journal of Health Education, November/December 1993 Supplement, S-55-S-56.

listening to a teacher talk about epidemics, from discussing peer pressure? It's the difference between reading about an ice cream cone and eating one. It's learning with the gut, learning from experience, even if the experience is a facsimile.

Optimally we all learn best when the subject matter applies to us personally. How many of us remember the formula for quadratic equations? or the capital of Sri Lanka? or the year that Justinian ascended to the throne of the Byzantine Empire? But we do remember how to drive a car, we do remember the capital of the state we live in, and we do remember the year of our birth (some of us with prodding).

Making a curriculum meaningful to students requires four things:

(1) knowing students—what they like, how they live, what they think about

(2) knowing the curriculum—primarily what it's designed to do

(3) varying teaching strategies—visual, auditory, kinesthetic, and combinations of these

(4) motivating students—encouraging them to make the curriculum meaningful to themselves.

How to Teach It

Here's how to do your own "Invisible Thread." You'll need about 30 sets of cards, seven per student, plus one set of larger masters for the teacher, attractive enough to motivate students to get more. Write a number in the upper right-hand corner of each set of cards (seven 1s, seven 2s, etc.). You'll also need a ball of yarn.

(1) Distribute one set of seven cards to each student. Have students take out a sheet of paper and number it from one to 30 (or the number of students there are in the room).

(2) Tell students that some of the symbols on the cards stand for good things and some of them stand for bad things. Say that when you give a signal, they can switch any one of the cards with any one of someone else's cards. Add that they don't have to switch at all, but when you say "Decide," they'll have 10 seconds to decide whether or not to switch.

(3) Tell students that once they switch, they should notice the number in the upper right-hand corner and write on their sheet of paper the name of the person who gave them the card next to the number of the card.

(4) Give student about 10 opportunities to switch, repeating the directions on occasion and reminding students that it's their choice whether or not to switch.

(5) After all students are back in their seats, choose one of the cards from your master set and hold it up. Say that the card stands for "happiness," and ask how many people either have the card in their hands right now or had it pass through their hands. Use the yarn to trace the route back to the person who was originally given the card.

(6) Repeat the process with "chicken pox" and then with "the AIDS virus."

(7) Ask students to draw parallels between the activity and some of the factors influencing the transmission and spread of HIV.

Obviously, this activity cannot stand alone. It serves as a provocative introductory lesson, however, for a unit on sexually transmitted diseases. It should be supported with current and accurate information on the topic.

What Else You Can Do

For some curricula, e.g, AIDS prevention or drug education curricula, personal impact is essential; it's the key motivator enabling students to learn. That's the bottom line for teachers: How can I get my students to learn? It's not enough to put food before a person; you've got to make the person want to eat it.

Think about what you can do in your classroom to bring that personal impact to each of your students: What do your students care about What do they like to do? Use examples from their lives, examples that they generate. Have them role-play. Have them create something, a story, a mural, a song, a game, a lesson. When it comes from *them*, they'll buy into the message. It will have *impact*.

AIDS EDUCATION: AN INTERDISCIPLINARY APPROACH BETWEEN THE HEALTH CARE PROFESSIONAL AND THE TEACHER OF THE DEAF†

Acquired Immune Deficiency Syndrome (AIDS) resulting from the Human Immunodeficiency Virus (HIV) is killing our youth, both hearing and deaf. Growing numbers of identified AIDS and HIV cases in the United States are forcing professionals in the fields of health care, education, and deaf education to interact in ways never before deemed necessary. This article addresses ways that health care professionals interact with teachers of deaf children. Good health habits and quality health education regarding AIDS and HIV infection, hopefully, will result.

How to Begin the Program

Starting an AIDS/HIV unit for deaf youths is not easy. The health care professional must consider several factors. First, deaf students have weak background knowledge in science, sex education (Fitz-Gerald, Fitz-Gerald, & Williams, 1978), and AIDS/HIV related issues. Second, deaf students have weak English language skills. For example, deaf adolescents read at the 3rd to 4th grade level (Allen, 1986; King & Quigley, 1985; Quigley & Paul, 1986, 1989, as cited in Paul & Quigley, 1990).

Third, unfortunately, myths and ignorance concerning sex and AIDS/HIV run rampant through school-aged deaf children. This ignorance is a result of a lack of information about AIDS among parents, guardians, and teachers, a lack of sex education and sexuality classes in schools, and poor communication skills between parents, teachers, and deaf children. Health care professionals working with parents, teachers, and school administrators can help remediate the ignorance by providing background information in classes, workshops and meetings for students, teachers, and parents. By using an American Sign Language (ASL) interpreter, the health care professional can more effectively teach AIDS/HIV information to deaf students.

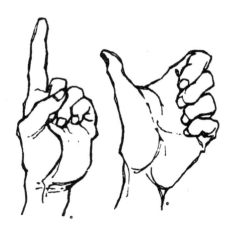

Presenting the Lesson

Limited background knowledge. Presenting a lesson to a class of deaf children requires that the presenter utilize a variety of educational approaches and techniques. Paramount is consideration of the information level to be presented and the background knowledge of the audience. Background knowledge about sex and sexuality for deaf children is considerably less than for hearing children. Why? Hearing children can learn about sex incidentally through television, radio, and conversations with their peers. Deafness closes off avenues for incidental learning and the deaf youth is often at a disadvantage in learning about sexuality issues. Additionally, deaf youth have fewer opportunities to discuss sexuality with their parents because of communication problems in the house. For example, a hearing child may overhear an Oprah Winfrey talk show on AIDS/HIV with the resulting discussion and discuss this subject with his or her

†By Gabriel A. Martin, Assistant Professor of Deaf Education at the Speech and Nursing Clinic, Lamar University, Beaumont, TX. This article was previously published in the Journal of Health Education, November/December 1993, 24(6), 374-375.

parents, while the deaf youth is not able to understand the topic or to communicate questions to the parents.

Language differences. The most important element that the health professional faces is that of language differences with the deaf children. Deaf children typically are bilingual, that is, they use some form of sign language and are learning English. Consequently, the presenter must offer his information with simple sentences in English using a sign language interpreter. At all times, the presenter must make sure that the deaf student understands the technical vocabulary contained in an AIDS/HIV lesson.

As a result of this language difference, health care professionals will find themselves in the unfamiliar and somewhat frightening situation of using an ASL interpreter. An ASL interpreter is one who has developed expressive and receptive skills in American Sign Language (ASL), follows a code of ethics, and interacts with deaf adults and children in their community to have a familiarity with their cultures. The sign language interpreter also will have skills in other sign systems for the purpose of communicating with a wide variety of deaf individuals who have varied communication levels.

The health care professional should remember four elements that will ease tension of the new situation. First, speak to the audience and not to the interpreter. The health care professional should face the deaf students because they are the ones receiving the information, not the interpreter. Second, speak at a normal rate of speed. The health care professional should avoid the tendency to say a few words and wait for the interpreter to catch-up. Third, speak clearly, distinctly, and avoid exaggeration of lip movements and facial expressions. This will ensure that deaf students have an opportunity to receive facial information. Finally, the experience of a time lag when asking questions and receiving a response is a result of interpreting one language (English) into another (ASL).

Multipresentation modes. The most common approach to presenting a topic is through the lecture mode. This traditional approach can be enhanced by utilizing visual displays to support the lecture (i.e., posters, bulletin boards, overhead projectors, movies). The more the health professional can make the presentation visual, the better it will be for hearing-impaired students because they are visual learners. One word of caution is that all the visual displays should represent the information at the appropriate level for the audience. Do not make the posters, bulletin boards, and overhead transparencies too childish for junior high school or high school, nor too abstract for preschool and elementary level. Further, all visual displays should be clear, neat, and accurate.

A second approach utilized with hearing-impaired classrooms is "role playing." This approach adds variety and excitement to any topic. Having students play parts enhances internalization of the concepts presented. It also personalizes learning and promotes a pragmatic connection of the facts. Integrating the lecture and "role playing" approaches greatly facilitates the student's learning. An example is where the health professional provides information about how one acquires AIDS/HIV, then has a pair of students "role play" a scenario where an individual (student 1) tells a friend (student 2) that he (student 1) is homosexual and the friend (student 2) becomes very angry because he (student 2) believes that both of them have AIDS/HIV infection because they are friends. The class then is given the opportunity to discuss this scenario with the presenter and the teacher. The scenario should be utilized at an appropriate grade level and maturity level for the class.

A final approach suggested is use of varied project activities designed to incorporate the information presented into a practical utilization in the real world. One example might be that students organize an AIDS Education Week program under sponsorship of the school. Students would develop and present "skits" and posters, and invite local community medical experts to lecture to the entire student body and faculty members. This also could be open to the public. Students learn how to organize a program, they learn how to involve the school and community, they learn to work as a team, and they incorporate the facts they learned about AIDS/HIV into a real world active project.

The three approaches above should not be considered as the only ones available. They represent the concept of providing the information to school-aged children from a variety of activities. These activities support and reinforce the internalization of factual information. A point to be mentioned here is that use of manipulatives (i.e., worksheets, stories, objects) helps to support the approaches discussed in the preceding paragraphs. Multi-sensory manipulations provide deeper levels of comprehension and internalization of concepts than do uni-sensory approaches.

Utilizing an interdisciplinary approach requires some education on the part of the health care professional as well as the classroom teacher of the hearing impaired. There is the need to share information and skills by both professionals. Both professionals utilize interpersonal skills to provide effective teaching. Each must rely on the other's strengths to provide an efficient and effective learning environment. There are several techniques and skills required of some health care professionals that may not have been developed or experienced previously. These include utilization of sign language interpreters, lesson presentations, language levels of hearing-impaired students, and classroom environment.

Conclusion

The need for AIDS/HIV education in the classroom is paramount for the hearing-impaired student. Because of the difficulty in the communication process and incorporation of a second language (ASL), the health care professional and the teacher of the deaf need to work in an interdisciplinary approach. In this manner, education about an issue that is highly controversial optimally may subdue the fears experienced by the community and will assist in providing much needed education to reverse the epidemic trend.

References

Allen, T. E. (1986). Patterns of academic achievement among hearing-impaired students: 1974 and 1983. In A. N. Schildroth & M. A. Karchmer (Eds.) . *Deaf children in America* (pp. 161-206). San Diego: College-Hill Press.

Fitz-Gerald, D., Fitz-Gerald, M., & Williams, C. M. (1978). The sex educator: Who's teaching the teacher sex education? *American Annals of the Deaf, 123*(1), 68-72.

King C., & Quigley, S. (1985). *Reading and deafness.* San Diego, CA: College-Hill.

Paul, P. V., & Quigley, S. P. (1990). *Education and deafness.* New York: Longman.

■

AIDS/HIV TEACHING IDEAS†

AIDS/HIV education is essential for the understanding and prevention of the disease. AIDS/HIV is a complex issue and thus demands a multifaceted approach. The condition may be viewed as a disease issue, a decision-making issue, a sexuality issue, and a death and dying issue.

A series of four teaching ideas are presented as they address each of the AIDS/HIV issues. The teaching techniques are as follows:

1. "Understanding AIDS/HIV"—a disease issue
2. "Who Do You Trust?"—a decision-making issue
3. "A Safer Sex Continuum"—a sexuality issue
4. "The Living Years"—a death and dying issue

Activity #1:
"Understanding AIDS/HIV"

Objective: After the bag demonstration, the student will be able to describe how HIV breaks down the immune system to allow the development of AIDS.

---

†By Barbara Beier, J. Leslie Oganowski, Richard A. Detert, and Kenneth Becker, members of the faculty at the University of Wisconsin-LaCrosse. This article was previously published in the Journal of Health Education, January/February 1993, 24(1), 47-49.

Preparation: Prepare envelopes for each student with the following shapes representing parts of the blood involved in the immune system. Place the HIV in only three of the envelopes.

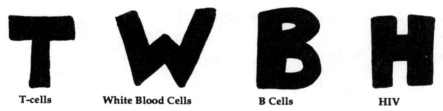

| T-cells | White Blood Cells | B Cells | HIV |

Necessary Materials:

    1 lunch-size paper bag for each student
    2 lunch-size bags for teacher demonstration
    markers or crayons
    prepared envelope for each student

Activity:

1. Instruct the students to color or decorate their bag to represent the skin.

2. Review the steps that take place when a germ enters the body by having each student put parts of the blood (from their envelope) in the bag. The teacher demonstrates by placing in the bag each cell type and explaining the action; i.e., white blood cells rush to the place where germs enter and attach to the germ to make it less dangerous to the person.

3. Introduce the functions of the immune system. A healthy immune system works to destroy nearly all types of germs, including many bacteria and viruses.

4. Write "immune" on the board. Have a student tell what is meant when someone says he/she is "immune" to something (protected/safe).

5. Conduct the following demonstration of the activities of the immune system in fighting germs.

    a. Hold two bags to represent the skin as a barrier to keep germs out. As long as the skin remains uninjured, it holds what's inside the body in and keeps the rest safely out.

    b. Reveal a break in the skin by tearing part of one bag. Have students name ways a break could occur (cuts, scratches, burns, scrapes, broken bones, surgery, intravenous drugs, ear piercing, tattoos, punctures).

    c. Toss some objects into the bags representing foreign bacteria, viruses, or germs. Explain that our blood contains white blood cells that fight germs. One kind of white blood cell (macrophage) moves through the blood and tissues to surround and "eat" germs. Toss some macrophage cells into the bag.

    d. T-cells are another type of white blood cell that help fight germs. T-cells attack and destroy viruses. Add T-cells to the bag. Stress that some T-cells serve as "command centers" for the body's battle against germs.

    e. Another kind of white blood cell is called a B-cell. Add the B-cells to the bag. B-cells produce chemicals called antibodies. Explain that antibodies can destroy viruses and other germs.

    f. Explain that some antibodies, even after destroying some germs, stay in the body to protect in case there is another exposure to the same type of germ. That is immunity.

    g. Ask students "What happens when the 'command center' in a real battle is destroyed?" Conclude that when germs attack the white blood cells (T-cells) that control the body's immune system, they can cripple the body's ability to fight off infection and disease.

    h. Ask who has an "H" in his/her envelope. Toss the "H" into the bag. This represents an HIV condition. AIDS is caused by a virus called HIV (human immunodeficiency virus). HIV destroys the "command centers" (T-cells) of the immune system and the body cannot fight off certain infections.

    i. The person with HIV does not usually die of HIV infection directly—the person with AIDS usually dies from other diseases that the body can no longer fight off.

Time Frame: The bag activity itself can be completed in a 30-40 minute class period. The preparatory information could take one class period to the activity. Questions about symptoms of HIV, children with HIV, and feelings associated with having an "H" in his/her bag could take varying amounts of time.

Do discuss with the class the chances of "having an HIV in his/her bag" and the risks of infection. Include a discussion of caring for the feelings of people who are infected.

Activity #2:
"Who Do You Trust?"

Objective: At the completion of this activity, students will be able to discuss the benefits and consequences of taking risks.

Preparation: Before students enter the room, the teacher places objects inside each of four large brown paper bags: (bag #1 = one mouse trap that is not set; bag #2 = one small mouse trap that is set; bag #3 = one large rat trap that is set; bag #4 = one block of wood).
There is one block of wood on the corner of the table.

Necessary Materials:
    4 large brown paper bags numbered 1 to 4
    2 mouse traps
    1 large rat trap
    2 blocks of wood
    table

Activity:
1.   Ask for three volunteers to come forward who are willing to take a risk. Describe the risk as selecting one of the paper bags. Volunteers will be asked to blindly reach to the bottom of the bag and grab whatever is in it. If it is the block of wood like the one on the corner of the table, they will receive a designated amount of money.
2.   Ask for three volunteers who will assist the risk takers in their adventure. Instruct these volunteers to move to the other side of the room.
3.   One at a time, ask each of the three assistants to open each of the bags and look at the contents. Ask them to be expressionless as they view each of the bags. Then ask each of the assistants if there is a block of wood in at least one of the bags. Once verified, ask (one at a time) if he/she would be willing to take the risk of reaching blindly into one of the bags. Some will say no; some, yes.
4.   Ask each assistant to meet a risk taker and quietly whisper in his/her ear what was seen in the bags. Then instruct the risk taker to whisper the same message to one other person in the room. Once all three have additional information about the contents, ask each of the risk takers if he/she is still willing to take the risk. Those who say "no" can be seated; those who are still willing to continue remain standing.
5.   Provide some more information to the risk takers (and the rest of the class) by revealing the contents of bag #1. Then reveal the contents of bag #2 by unsetting the mouse trap with a folded piece of paper. Ask again which risk takers would still be willing to blindly reach into one of the two remaining bags.
6.   Ask the assistants to provide a bit more information to the risk takers and the rest of the class by asking whether a consequence of reaching into one of the bags could result in (a) pain, (b) broken fingers, or (c) the presence of blood? Then ask again who might be willing to take the risk.
7.   Teacher places remaining risk takers in the front of the room and asks them one more time if they are willing to take the risk. If yes, mix the bags up and ask the risk takers to turn around. By now, most risk takers have quit!
8.   Of course, the teacher stops the activity at this point as students could get injured if they actually reached into bag #3. The bag contents are now revealed.
9.   Follow-up discussion:
    a.   Ask the risk takers to tell the group what their assistant whispered in their ear.
    b.   Did all the assistants see the same contents?
    c.   Discuss how the risk takers thought they could "beat the odds."
    d.   Discuss comments that encouraged/discouraged each from stopping or continuing with the activity.
    e.   Finally, discuss what risks each are willing to take; which would not be safe risks; what risks are involved with AIDS/HIV conditions.

Time Frame: This activity takes between 20-40 minutes to complete. The time frame may vary depending on grade level and the number of comments made or points raised during the discussion.

Activity #3:
"A Safer Sex Continuum"

Objective: At the completion of this activity the student will be able to identify means of transmission of AIDS/HIV on a safer to unsafe continuum.

Preparation: When discussing the issue of AIDS in the classroom, one way to introduce safe and unsafe sexual practices is by using the "Safer Sex Continuum." This activity would be part of a larger unit on sexuality or sexually transmitted diseases (STDs) and would be utilized once the students had developed a degree of comfort in discussing sexual topics.

Materials Necessary:
    chalkboard and chalk
    (or newsprint and marking pens)

Activity:
    1.   Introduce the topic by having students consider the methods of transmission of the HIV virus and sexual practices. Place the continuum shown at the bottom of the page on the chalkboard.
    2.   At this point, ask the students to "place" a sexual activity on this continuum on the appropriate position so as to indicate the "safeness" or "riskiness" of the behavior. As each behavior or sexual activity is suggested, the elements involved in ranking that behavior in that position should also be discussed. This method involves the students in analyzing each sexual activity based upon their knowledge of the transmission of the HIV virus. It is also a method that could be useful in introducing sensitive topics such as masturbation, condom use, and anal intercourse.
    3.   Clarification of certain activities is a productive outcome of this activity if students are allowed to engage in open discussion and ask questions. For instance, one popular misconception discovered with this approach was that some students considered a sexual monogamous relationship to mean having sex with "one person at a time."

Time Frame: This activity takes between 30 and 50 minutes to complete depending upon (1) the level of knowledge of the students, (2) the degree of comfort with discussing sexual topics, and (3) the amount of discussion time allowed.

Activity #4:
"The Living Years"

Objective: At the completion of this activity, the student will be able to verbalize his/her reactions to AIDS as a death and dying issue.

Preparation: One effective way we found to address AIDS as a death and dying issue was to play a song that many students may have heard on popular hit radio stations. "The Living Years," recorded by Mike and the Mechanics, was played and students were encouraged to follow along with the printed words. Introductory statements may include: "Think about the words and what they say about death and dying," or, "As you listen to the words of this song, think about your thoughts on death, dying, and AIDS."

Materials Necessary:
    tape: "The Living Years," by Mike and the Mechanics
    printed words to the song
    tape player

The Living Years

Every generation
Blames the one before
And all of their frustrations
Come beating in your door.

I know that I'm a prisoner
To all my father held so dear
I know that I'm a hostage
To all his hopes and fears
I just wish I could have told him
In the living years.

Crumpled bits of paper
Filled with imperfect thought
Stilted conversations
I'm afraid that's all we've got.

You say you just don't see it

He says it's perfect sense
You just can't get agreement
In this present tense
We all talk a different language
Talking in defense.

Say it loud, say it clear
You can listen as well as you hear
It's too late when we die
To admit we don't see eye to eye.

So we open up in quarrel
Between the present and the past
We only sacrifice the future

It's the bitterness that lasts.
So don't yield to the fortunes
You sometimes see as fate
It may have a new perspective
On a different day
And if you don't give up,
And don't give in
You may just be OK.

Say it loud, say it clear
You can listen as well as you hear
It's too late when we die
To admit we don't see eye to eye.

I wasn't there that morning
When my father passed away
I didn't get to tell him
All the things I had to say,
I think I caught his spirit
Later that same year
I'm sure I heard his echo
In my baby's new born tears
I just wish I could have told him
In the living years.

"The Living Years," Mike and the Mechanics (1988), Atlantic Record Corporation, 75 Rockefeller Plaza, New York, NY 10019.

PARENT EDUCATION

DISCIPLINE: A PARENTING DILEMMA†

The philosophical continuum of parental discipline ranges from "child abuse" on one extreme to "passive acceptance of the child's unmanageable behavior" on the other. Repercussions to disciplinary actions are both positive and negative and affect both child and parental health.

Attempting to apply specific disciplinary measures to correct a child's unacceptable behavior can often be a matter of trial and error. For each couple experiencing parenthood, there will be frustration and aggravation as well as love and delight.

Parents admittedly make mistakes in their administration of discipline. Today the effectiveness of the traditional method of corporal punishment is much in doubt. It is through this method that children quickly learn "might means right." Since there are seldom any academic classes addressing the problems of parenting, we are often left with past disciplinary experiences as our only legacy of such skills.

The selection of behavioral management techniques by a parent depends on the child's overt behavior which is interfering with parental rules or guidelines.

Behavioral management is basically a set of procedures that, when appropriately applied, usually decrease undesirable behavior and hopefully increase desirable behavior. These parental procedures require experience and practice to be successful. Punishment is defined as administering an aversive consequence or withdrawing positive reinforcement in order to reduce the possibility of the recurrence of a task or demonstration of a maladaptive behavior (Azrin & Holz, 1966).

Discipline is a state of order based upon rules and regulations. In its simplest terms, it is teaching people to follow specific rules.

There is a major difference between punishment and discipline, however. In punishment, pain follows an act that someone else disapproves of, and the someone else usually provides the pain. With discipline, the pain is a natural and realistic consequence of a person's behavior. Unlike punishment, discipline is rarely arbitrary; it asks that a child evaluate his behavior and commit himself to a better course of action (Glasser, 1965).

Preventive behavioral management is the best approach to parenting. Management guidelines need to be established early and explained in detail, along with possible consequences as a result of violating these guidelines.

The importance of parent-child communication is paramount in the prevention-behavior management continuum. Being able to discuss fully problems, potential crises, and the providing of parental support, can perhaps reduce the probability of future behavioral problems.

Health problems pertaining to mental health, sexuality, mood modifiers, nutrition and other related areas often center around a poor self-concept or self-esteem. If potential parents realize the importance of the development of their child's self-concept and facilitate open, two-way communication, discipline techniques will be more easily understood and tolerated.

---

†By Patrick K. Tow, Associate Professor of Health Education, Department of Health, Physical Education and Recreation, Old Dominion University, Norfolk, VA, and Warren L. McNab, Associate Professor of Health Education, School of Health, Physical Education, Recreation and Dance, University of Nevada, Las Vegas, NV. This article was previously published in Health Education, February/March 1985, 16(1), 45-47.

The positive or negative development of the child depends on the parental attitudes, values, and discipline philosophy which many times emulates the positive or negative relationship they experienced with their own parents.

Glasser (1965) suggests parents take the following steps in addressing behavioral problems:

1. Ask the child if what he/she did was against your parental rules.
2. Ask the child to evaluate himself as to the reason behind his/her actions or behavior.
3. Collectively the parent(s) and the child should devise a plan and commitment to do better.
4. As a parent, explain you will not accept anything but a change in behavior.
5. Otherwise, specific consequences of breaking the rules will be enforced. In following these steps, parents should build on the positive strengths of their children, control emotions, and facilitate positive communication.

The Role of Health Education

Educational methodologies which allow parents or prospective parents hypothetically to recognize potential problem areas, establish guidelines in disciplining children, and practice the communication techniques which enhance the behavioral management procedure, certainly would be beneficial. Prospective parents are not prepared, nor do they realize what parental responsibilities encompass. Education for parenthood segments of health education courses should involve a variety of methodologies geared toward the prevention, management, and communication skills needed to cope with specific behavior problems.

In professional preparation programs, health educators should provide numerous methodologies to students involving disciplinary measures. Following is a procedure that has been successful in providing students in health education with parental behavioral management experience.

Step 1. Identify Discipline Alternatives

Chances are that students in your class have had first-hand experience with a variety of disciplinary measures employed by their own parents. Tap into this valuable resource at your disposal. Depend upon their past encounters to help shape the preliminary portion of the strategy by encouraging them to identify a list of these measures.

After the brainstorming session, carry out a class tally of the number of students having experience in each of the measures listed. This will help students realize there is a commonality, though no absolute uniformity, in discipline practices among parents. It also allows students the opportunity to see there are many different and perhaps more effective ways to handle disciplinary problems. This list usually includes the following disciplinary alternatives:

1. Corporal punishment (i.e., use of physical force).
2. Total loss of privileges (e.g., no TV, music, or parties).
3. Home detention (i.e., grounded at home for a period of time; room confinement).
4. Fines (i.e., suspension or reduced allowance; pay a penalty).
5. Assignment of extra household duties (i.e., additional chores on top of regular duties).
6. Verbal put-downs (i.e., belittle or scold).
7. Curbing of privileges (e.g., earlier curfew, restrictions).
8. Ignoring the problem (i.e., pay little or no attention to the child).

No doubt there are proponents and opponents to one or more of these disciplinary techniques. Part of this step requires students to provide advantages and disadvantages for each of the measures cited.

Step 2. Examine Potential Disciplinary Problems

After identifying specific disciplinary alternatives, the types of problems confronted by new parents over the years should be identified. After all, our society would like to believe its members designate appropriate "punishment" tailored to the nature of the "crime" committed. Presumably the same logic would apply to the disciplinary problems created by children in a family. This second step requires students to list problems frequently encountered at home for which disciplinary measures may be applied. Examples of some potential disciplinary problems would probably include:

1. Talking back or "sassing"
2. Excessive TV watching
3. Use of profanity
4. Staying out late without checking in
5. Lying
6. Shoplifting
7. Fighting with peers
8. Playing with matches
9. Crossing streets without adult supervision
10. Smoking cigarettes
11. Coming home drunk
12. Stealing money from parents
13. Crying or refusing to leave toy or candy section of store
14. Horseplay leading to property damage
15. Cheating at school
16. Accepting treats from strangers
17. Neglecting household chores
18. Looking through pornographic materials
19. Playing hooky from school
20. Running away from home
21. Eating snacks before meals
22. Drunk while driving
23. Crying or refusing to visit doctor's or dentist's office
24. Smoking marijuana
25. Repeat traffic law offender
26. Premarital pregnancy experienced by daughter or caused by son
27. Violation of curfew on weekday or weekend
28. Hitting the parent in anger
29. Hanging around with bad company
30. Failing academically at school

As one can easily surmise from this partial listing of disciplinary problems, some are major concerns while others do not need redress of any kind. Yet many parents have a way of misconstruing a wide assortment of concerns as being a personal matter deserving punitive action. One also sees that some concerns can be handled differently with a young child than with a teenager.

Step 3. Examine Specific Circumstances and Determine a Reasonable Course of Disciplinary Action

This step requires students in the class to be paired off in couples simulating two parents.

Ask the prospective parents to examine each of the situations listed and determine whether it truly constitutes a bonafide disciplinary problem. The parents are then to determine the proper disciplinary action, if any, to be applied to each of the problems listed earlier. It must be stressed to these pseudo-parents that concurrence should exist between them on the final decision. This exercise can also be done individually to symbolize the single parent family.

Step 4. Evaluation and Discussion of the Disciplinary Decision

The last step of this strategy involves convening the class to listen collectively to and discuss similar or different ways these prospective parents would handle such disciplinary problems in their own families. The opportunity to discuss the reasons for variations in approaching the same disciplinary problems should be provided.

Summary

The positive familial relationship can be an extremely rewarding and enjoyable experience. The key, perhaps, is understanding the magnitude of the responsibility of parenthood, the preparation of the predictable, and coping with the unpredictable behavioral management difficulties that one may encounter as a parent.

Even before anticipating a pregnancy, prospective parents should evaluate the needs and goals they hope to satisfy by having children. Every child should be a wanted child. In having children, parents should feel a sense of creative accomplishment in guiding and helping a child grow into a well-functioning adult. The parent is the most important teacher the child will ever have. Helping their children through behavior management in developing positive physical, mental, intellectual, and social adjustments in life can be a wonderfully rewarding experience for parents. Even the best parents make mistakes, but with proper knowledge, planning, and discipline experience, they can overcome many of the difficulties of child-rearing. Good parents will evaluate the discipline situation and respect the child as an individual, satisfy the psychological and behavioral needs of the child, and provide the child with emotional security, sympathy, and understanding.

In the majority of school systems, parenting and behavioral management skills are not included in the health curriculum. There is a definite need for cognitive and effective teachings regarding the behavioral management of children. The objective is to provide as many relevant and realistic experiences as possible to inform students, as potential parents, of the responsibilities in preparing for parenthood.

There is a need to dispel the unrealistic notion that as future parents they will rear perfectly obedient children. Disciplinary measures come in many forms—held in disdain by some and strongly endorsed by others. Effective experimental behavioral management techniques encourage effective parent-child communication skills through listening, critical thinking, and assertiveness.

Health programs which include parental discipline techniques can provide assistance to young people to prepare for parenthood, reduce certain predictable health problems, and hopefully enhance the overall health of the child and parent in the process.

References

Azrin, N. H., & Holz, O. C. (1966). Punishment, in W. K. Honig (Ed.). *Operant behavior areas of research and application.* New York: Appleton-Century-Crofts.

Glasser, W. (1965). *Reality therapy.* New York: Harper & Row.

PARENT/CAREGIVER HEALTH EDUCATION IN THE DAYCARE CENTER†

Infants and young children represent the most dependent segment of our society. They rely totally on their parents and caregivers ("Caregiver" refers to the individual responsible for the child while the parent is away, for example, due to employment outside the home) to meet their basic needs, provide a caring environment, and protect them from injury and harm. Parents and caregivers want to be familiar with all information related to the health and safety of their young children, but many individuals feel they lack sufficient knowledge in all areas such as basic child care, safety and first aid, and nutrition. The individual may experience feelings of guilt or lack of confidence if the child develops a preventable illness or is injured. Acquisition of this information can be another source of frustration. Parents and caregivers have a natural interest in their child's well-being and they ask questions of one another to meet their child's needs. Examples of health/safety related questions which one might expect are (parent to doctor) "What immunizations are recommended?"; (parent to caregiver) "Are the electrical outlets properly covered and are toys appropriate for the child's age?" or (caregiver to parent) "Your child seems unusually tired. Has he/she been ill or had any fever?". Questions such as these are essential to optimal

†By Charlotte M. Hendricks, Health Educator and Special Projects Coordinator, JCCEO Headstart, Birmingham, AL. This article was previously published in Health Education, September/October 1990, 21(5), 56-57.

child care, but parents and caregivers may not realize their importance. Therefore, one goal of health education for this population is to increase awareness of health related issues and the importance of healthy behaviors. Caregivers then can be directed to further sources of information.

Daycare centers are seldom the target of formal health education programs. This is a serious problem when one considers the growing number of children enrolled in such programs. More than half of all pre-school age children have employed mothers (the traditional caregiver) and about half these mothers use some form of day care (American Academy of Pediatrics, 1987). Unfortunately, parents and caregivers of young children in daycare programs often cannot arrange time to participate in a structured health education program at the center. Parents have diverse schedules, so it is difficult to schedule a time convenient for each. Daycare staff are limited to the time before and after work hours for educational programs, creating additional scheduling difficulty since many daycare staff work on individualized schedules rather than on standard shifts. For such reasons, parents and caregivers require effortless access to concise information that has immediate application to their child's developmental or health needs.

Health education may occur only through efforts of a concerned parent or caregiver familiar with the hectic schedules of other parents and caregivers. The purpose of this article is to describe a health education program which can be implemented easily in a daycare center by any individual with the proper interest and motivation, and does not require a trained health educator.

The first component involves placing colorful, informative posters by each outer door. Parents and caregivers can read the information as they take their child to or from the center. The primary purpose of the poster is to make individuals aware of the topic. Thus, the key to success is color and design. The poster must be visually appealing to *both* children and adults and must attract their attention. A different poster and topic is presented each month.

The second component provides further information related to the topic through pamphlets and brochures that the individual can keep for future reference. A colorful box containing copies of the material is placed near the poster. As with posters, material are changed monthly.

The difficulty in conducting this program may be to locate appropriate (and free) posters and pamphlets. Many available health education posters are related to adolescent and adult topics rather than childhood health issues. Few health education printed materials relate specifically to the health and safety needs of young children. This lack of appropriate materials can affect greatly the impact of a health education program. If parents perceive materials (such as stop smoking or cardiovascular disease information) to be unrelated to their child's immediate needs, they may ignore future materials. Also, selected materials must be carefully reviewed for accuracy, readability, and suitability of information. This will require expertise of an individual trained in health education and/or a related profession.

Likely sources of appropriate materials may include companies that market children's toys, infant formula/foods, medicines, diapers, or clothing. Professional or governmental organizations such as the American Academy of Pediatrics, the National Highway Traffic Safety Commission, the National Institute of Dental Research, and the Consumer Product Safety Commission have materials at little or no cost. Voluntary and public health organizations, such as the American Heart Association the American Lung Association, and local Children's Hospitals also provide excellent materials.

The need for immediate application of information is met through the third component, presentation of weekly "Health Tips," or "Health Questions." A sheet of colored paper is folded in half and fastened to a bulletin board or other prepared surface. The question is printed on the outside flap, preferably along with clip-art or a picture to attract the individual's attention. The person must then open the folded paper to read the answer or health tip. Since this information is changed weekly, it serves either to highlight information in the related pamphlet or to provide up-to-date information about current health events. For example, a question might ask "What food most often causes choking?" Answer: "Hot dogs. Other foods that young children should not eat are hard candies, Vienna sausages, grapes, and nuts." Another topic area for which a question could be asked might be based on news coverage of pesticide contamination of apple products.

The fourth component of this program may be maintenance of an on-site library including books and videocassettes. Parents themselves may be the best source of material since many are willing to share their personal books and videotapes. Also, the sources mentioned earlier may provide single copies of books or videotapes or may provide copyright permission for their videotaped materials. If an on-site library is not feasible, a reference list of materials available at the local public library can be provided.

The final element to a successful health education program is listening to participants. Parents and caregivers can suggest topics and ask questions to make the program more interesting and applicable. The comments may be collected by providing paper, pencil, and a drop box, or have parents inform their child's teacher of their interests.

This entire program can be directed by an individual parent or caregiver, or the program director may choose to coordinate the activities and delegate responsibilities to interested parents and caregivers. A few simple steps such as these can not only make a great difference in the adults' confidence and security as they care for their child, but can also help create a healthy, happy, and safe childhood.

Reference

American Academy of Pediatrics. (1987, February 15). *News release.* Elk Grove Village, IL.

PROGRAM AND
INSTRUCTIONAL RESOURCES

Ellen Candles, drug prevention coordinator for a mid-size school district in Wisconsin, sits behind a desk watching the veins on a young woman's neck become more and more pronounced even as her voice maintains a calm, determined tone. The woman's son is in the fourth grade, and she is describing the drug education program he is being taught:

". . . school is not a place for psychotherapy. I do not pay taxes for my son to feel that he has to tell family secrets in order to pass this class. My son has strong values, and I don't want them subverted by a curriculum that turns children against their parents and pries into their personal lives."

Ms. Candles nods as the woman continues with claims that the curriculum espouses New Age philosophy, promotes drug use, reflects values clarification, and violates the Hatch Act. The woman concludes by demanding not only that her son be removed from the drug education class, but also that the curriculum be removed from the district's program.

The following week, the woman, along with five other parents, will take her complaints to the School Board. These parents will be adamant, persistent, and organized.

This is not an uncommon scenario—in any state, in any community. Drug education programs, *health* programs, are constantly being challenged, sometimes by well-meaning parents with legitimate concerns about what their children are learning in school, sometimes by fanatics of the right whose sole agenda is to make everyone adapt to their narrow, intolerant beliefs, and everything in between. To the extent that you can distinguish people's motives, you'll better serve the interests of your students and your district.

People who rant about the devil's exerting influence over the developers of a curriculum may be subjects for amusing anecdotes, but their impact has been serious and far-reaching. The right is organized, well-funded, and single-minded. We need to address their concerns as much as anyone's, but there are certain points to remember if we are to address their concerns successfully. Here are some:

(1) Know your rules and your allies. First, know the process by which curricula are adopted in your district. Understand how the system works so you can guarantee that no one is stampeded into making a decision based on an emotional presentation. Second, know your allies. Rely on others for support, for information, and for ideas. Establish alliances and conditions to support your health education program.

(2) Determine whether the challengers in fact live in your district or have children in your district's schools. This, of course, goes to the heart of their concerns; it may have nothing to do with their own children, but more to do with a national political agenda.

(3) Ask them to document their concerns in writing. Having a concern in writing accomplishes several objectives: it makes the person adhere to a consistent line; it makes the person be specific, so you

---

†*By Neal Starkman, writer and developer, and Jerry Warren, Health Education Specialist, at Comprehensive Health Education Foundation, Seattle, WA. This article was previously published in the Journal of Health Education, November/December 1993 Supplement, S-50-S-51.*

in turn can be specific in your response; it enables you to refer the concern to others, without fear of mis-interpretation.

(4) Ask challengers if they personally have read the material in question. Sometimes people will merely repeat a rumor they've heard rather than examine the material in context. Offer to show the material in question.

(5) Ask for definitions of terms, e.g., "sensitivity training," "secular humanism." Quite often people use terms to generate emotion rather than reason; they really don't know what "sensitivity training" or "secular humanism" means. If you can get them to define their terms, it will be easier to reject their claims.

(6) Talk about the overall goals of the curriculum and the objectives of the lessons, not each word in each activity. A curriculum is complex. It includes not only written material, but also the teacher, the students, and the classroom environment. Targeting a word or sentence can lead people astray from the main thrust of the lesson and the program. You're better off if your curriculum is age-appropriate, is based on reliable research, and uses acceptable methodology.

(7) Keep in focus the needs of the students. Don't be shifted form the important issues. You're not in a position to debate the religious freedom of the parent or the moral decay of civilization or the lack of respect young people have for their elders. Presumably, you have a mandate to provide effective health education for your students. *That's* the issue.

(8) Stay positive. This could be the most difficult point to remember. Sometimes you're going to be interacting with hateful, spiteful people who care nothing for children, nothing for education, nothing for you. In these cases, you might have to accept a bottom line: *you won't be able to convince them of anything.* Arguing with logic is alien to some people, and you might as well agree to disagree. Be assured that you're doing what's right for children and what's consistent with the goals of your job.

This is tough work: It makes you expend time and energy on something that distracts you from what you want to be doing. It exposes you to intolerance and negativity when you'd prefer to be focusing on the promise and hope of health education. But remember: You're not alone. Most people don't agree with the fanatics. Most people support health education. These are the people you need to stand the ground with you.

Here are people who will stand the ground with you. Write to the following organizations if you're struggling with a challenge:

American Civil Liberties Union
132 West 43rd Street
New York, NY 10036
ATTN: Alan Reitman

Association for the Advancement
    of Health Education
1900 Association Drive
Reston, VA 22091
ATTN: Becky Smith

National School Health Education Coalition
1000 Vermont Avenue, NW, Suite 400
Washington, DC 20005
ATTN: Pat Cooper

American Library Association
Office of Intellectual Freedom
50 E. Huron Street
Chicago, IL 60611
ATTN: Judith Drug

Comprehensive Health Education Foundation
22323 Pacific Highway S.
Seattle, WA 98198
ATTN: Jerry Warren or Neal Starkman

People for the American Way
2000 M St., Suite 400
Washington, DC 20036
ATTN: Field Department

FOCUS GROUP DISCUSSIONS:
AN APPLICATION TO TEACHING†

The focus group interview is a small group discussion, guided by a moderator, to gain an understanding of participants' knowledge, attitudes, values, and perceptions of a particular topic. The group's composition and discussion are carefully planned to create a permissive, nonthreatening environment conducive to revelation and disclosure. Participants are encouraged to express differing perceptions, ask questions, and respond to comments of other participants, as well as to those presented by the moderator (Kreuger, 1989).

You probably have heard about use of focus group interviews in health education research. They have proven highly effective as a tool for "understanding and developing sensitivity toward those we serve" (Basch, 1987, p. 436). Less attention has been given to the important educational role that focus groups can play in helping participants clarify values, expand their knowledge, and motivate them to adopt healthy behaviors. This article looks at each of these applications, research, and education, as they may be used by school based health educators. We give special attention to curricula development and risk reduction, using smoking cessation as an example.

Understanding Student Perceptions

As a research tool, focus group interviews offer a relatively rapid and inexpensive way to gain an understanding of students' perceptions of a health topic such as smoking and smoking cessation curricula. The loosely structured discussion format is ideal for uncovering factors that influence students' decisions and the feelings associated with various views about the topic. Information that is especially valuable in determining the content, key messages, materials, and teaching methods which are needed to design risk reduction curricula effectively includes:

• **Knowledge**: What do they already know? What misinformation needs to be corrected? What do they want to know?

• **Perceptions**: What factors deter them from adopting healthy practices? What aspirations, interests, or other factors can be used to motivate them to adopt healthy practices?

• **Assessment of teaching techniques**: Which teaching methods do they enjoy the most? Which do they believe are most effective in helping them understand new information? Which do they find most effective in helping them change health behaviors?

• **Assessment of existing or proposed teaching materials**: Do they understand the information presented? What do they like and dislike about the content, illustrations, and format of the proposed materials. Do they find the spokesperson(s) credible and convincing? Do they find the message(s) persuasive?

A note of caution: in curricula development, results of focus group research usually are confirmed using a more structured survey that allows the health educator to assess the extent to which issues are shared by a larger group. It is important also to supplement data obtained from students with the views of other key groups, particularly parents, teachers, and community representatives.

Empowering Students to Adopt Healthy Behaviors

Although focus group discussions are conducted primarily to collect information, most participants find them highly educational, even empowering (Bryant & Bailey, 1990). This is not surprising. Small group processes have been used in health education since Kurt Lewin and Margaret Mead conducted group experiments during World War II. Using lectures and small group discussions, they found that

†By Carol Bryant, Assistant Professor, and Elizabeth Gulitz, Associate Professor, in the Department of Community and Family Health, College of Public Health, University of South Florida, Tampa, FL. This article was previously published in the Journal of Health Education, May/June 1993, 24(3), 188-189.

people are more likely to act on the knowledge that they have learned if they make a commitment in a group to do so, even if they know that they will never see other group members again (Basch, 1987).

Focus group discussions are especially valuable for health educators working with students. First, students learn a great deal from their peers. The safety of being with a group of other students provides an avenue for self-discovery, self-expression, and an opportunity to compare their views with those of their peers. The group interaction and camaraderie that typically develops within the group enhances students' abilities to uncover factors that influence their health decisions and stimulates a willingness to share these discoveries with others. Participants often gain the support from the group to express socially unpopular, embarrassing, or anxiety producing views. Also, most groups contain one or more courageous students who share information that others would prefer to withhold, thereby provoking the more timid respondents to make similar disclosures (Goldman & McDonald, 1987). In this way, focus group discussions encourage value clarification, and give students a rare opportunity to teach each other. This instills confidence and increases the likelihood that students will translate this new knowledge into behavioral change. In a discussion of smoking, for example, students may gain a new awareness of the many factors that influence their decision to smoke. They may learn for the first time that others share many of their concerns. For those voicing a public position against smoking, the group interaction reinforces their decision not to smoke.

Second, focus group interviews allow the health educator to observe respondents' interactions as they share feelings, form opinions, and influence each other, as they would in other social settings. If smokers and nonsmokers are mixed in a group, it is possible to assess the strength of their convictions as they defend their respective positions. How do smokers respond to the view that smokers are less attractive sexually because of bad breath and clothing? How do the nonsmokers counter the advantages of smoking?

During the course of group discussions, some students change their opinions or beliefs. Often, focus group participants are able to correct misinformation and encourage adoption of healthier behaviors without guidance of an educator or moderator. In addition to the impact the group interaction has on participants' views or behavior, the opportunity to observe the interaction enables the moderator to identify the comments or types of interaction that resulted in the shift. This also may provide information useful in designing educational messages, materials, and other aspects of risk reduction curricula.

Third, focus group interviews use a loosely structured interview format to present ideas or broad topics for discussion. Students as well as the moderator may initiate new topics and direct the conversation to areas not previously recognized as relevant. For instance, students are able to address their concerns about smoking and to present ideas for encouraging young people to quit that could not be anticipated by the moderator. This makes the group discussion effective as both an educational and research tool, generating insights that can be incorporated into other educational materials and messages.

Fourth, like people of all ages, students gain a sense of importance from participating in a project that will help others. Focus group discussions offer a rare opportunity to serve as expert, expressing views while one or more adults listen respectfully and intently. Moderators often are impressed with how articulate and intelligent people appear in focus groups compared to other settings in which their opinions are not as highly valued. They also note the large percentage of people who express gratitude for being included and ask to participate in future groups.

Special Challenges

Focus group discussions with students pose several challenges to the health educator. Because teens and pre-teens are easily influenced by their peers, the moderator should be skilled at eliciting divergent opinions and controlling the influence of more dominant, vocal participants. Examples include avoiding eye contact with a student who is doing most of the talking or looking directly at a more reticent group member when asking a question (KreuGer, 1989; Goldman & McDonald, 1987). The interview protocol can be designed to ensure that a balance of techniques also helps to counter peer pressure and to facilitate discussion of unpopular or embarrassing views, especially when working with a group of students who know each other. Examples include free association, story completion exercises, and photo sort exercises (Debus, 1989). In the photo sort exercise, students are given a set of photographs of teens representing a variety of class and ethnic groups and are asked to identify the people who would smoke and those who would not. As students discuss the reasons for their choices, they are likely to reveal subtle characteristics of smokers that otherwise would require unusual awareness and verbal skill. In the course of imagining the lives and attributes of these photographed teens, the students are likely to discover and disclose information about their own ideas and personalities.

In sum, focus group discussions offer the health educator working in school settings a valuable research method for gaining increased awareness of students' knowledge, attitudes, and perceptions of health topics, and an educational technique to empower them to adopt healthier lifestyles. For a more detailed discussion of the methodological issues involved in conducting and analyzing focus group research, consult Mary Debus' *Handbook for Excellence in Focus Group Research* (1989), Richard Kreuger's *Focus Groups: A Practical Guide for the Applied Researcher* (1989), and Alfred Goldman and Susan McDonald's *The Group Depth Interview: Principles and Practice* (1987).

References

Basch, C. (1987). Focus group interview: An underutilized research technique for improving theory and practice in health education. *Health Education Quarterly, 14*(4), 411-448.

Bryant, C., & Bailey, D. (1990) The use of focus groups in program development. *National Association of Practicing Anthropologists Bulletin (10),* 24-39.

Debus, M. (1989). *Handbook for excellence in focus group research.* Washington, DC: Academy for Educational Development.

Goldman, A., & McDonald, S. (1987). *The group depth interview.* New Jersey: Prentice-Hall, Inc.

Kreuger, R. (1989). *Focus groups: A practical guide for applied research.* California: Sage Publications.

COGNITIVE MAPPING:
AN ACTIVITY FOR HEALTH EDUCATION†

Health educators are in general agreement that health behavior is a decision-making process, where decisions are based on critical examination of possible alternatives (Pollock & Middleton, 1989). Teachers of health education, then, should be concerned with selecting and utilizing methods of teaching designed to assist students in developing problem-solving skills. An information processing approach to student learning offers a useful framework for thinking about process-centered teaching which can encourage reasoning and reflection, rather than recitation by students.

Current information processing approaches to learning assume that an individual constructs models of reality from interactions with the environment and these prototypes are stored as networks of related schemata or structures for future reference or interpretation (Shuell, 1986). It is the qualitative organization of this network that is as important as learning from an information processing perspective involving creation of cognitive structures which help students arrange knowledge in a meaningful way. Knowledge structures are based on the content of a particular course but are created individually by students. These internal cognitive representations are used to interpret new knowledge, forming the basis for problem solving. There is general agreement that in order for basic health content to be useful to students, the information acquired must represent more than a compilation of facts, laws, and theories to be memorized for a unit examination. If learning is to be a lifelong process enabling students to think and use cognitive skills for more healthful living, teachers must assist students in their development of more organized and elaborate cognitive structures.

---

†*By Jo A. Carter, Associate Professor of Health Education/Pedagogy, and Melinda A. Solmon, Assistant Professor of Pedagogy, Department of Kinesiology, Louisiana State University, Baton Rouge, LA. This article was previously published in the Journal of Health Education, March/April 1994, 25(2), 108-109.*

Description of the Mapping Activity

Construction of concept maps is the one way to measure students' knowledge structures and the process can be beneficial in helping students learn to think more analytically and productively in health education. First, the teacher asks each student to formulate a list of terms about a particular health topic or provides the student with a teacher-constructed list. The goal is for students to arrange the terms in some spatial way which represents their personal understanding of the content. Students are asked to draw a map or picture which displays their understanding of the content, using connecting lines to show relationships. A sample map prepared by the teacher on another topic may be used as an example. It is important to emphasize that there is no one correct way to display the terms. The objective is for each student to construct a network that makes sense to him or her. Since cognitive maps reflect the knowledge structure of a student, several useful applications can be offered for teachers.

The Process in Action

Assessment of Knowledge

Students construct a map prior to instruction so the depth and breadth of understanding about a topic can be determined. Figures 1 and 2 illustrate pretest maps showing two different levels of prior knowledge. The concept map can be used in lieu of or in addition to a pretest. As students progress through the unit, new maps should be generated to serve as indicators of learning and to identify areas of misunderstanding. Maps drawn during instruction can show content inadequacies (long vertical lists) or illogical associations(two totally unrelated concepts connected). The basis for gaps and inadequacies in comprehension of health content then can be studied and specific plans can be made to address misconceptions or limited understanding.

Organizing Content

Use an instructor-prepared map as a visual when introducing a topic. The map can function as a guide for sequencing content and can provide a vehicle for helping students link new ideas to what they already know. Identification of major concepts or principles can be used as advanced organizers and, as subconcepts are introduced, relationships can be explained while viewing the map. This helps students anchor new terminology to that previously learned.

Facilitating Comprehension

Students are asked to look at their maps during class, then form small groups to compare and discuss the maps. Student maps can be compared with the map constructed by the teacher. Discussion of differences shows students that content can be understood and interpreted in different ways, and that there is not always just one right answer. Comparison of the various networks can help students establish links between concepts which will improve comprehension. While simple recall of subject matter is important, development of higher level cognitive skills (analysis, synthesis) is necessary before information can be applied to problem-solving situations.

In summary, cognitive maps offer health education teachers a powerful teaching tool which can be useful to: (1) link new health concepts with prior health knowledge, (2) give direction for organizing and anchoring new health information, (3) help students integrate and synthesize health concepts and subconcepts holistically, both within and between the designated health content areas, and (4) provide the teacher with opportunities to help students develop cognitive skills needed for critical thinking and problem solving. Mapping is simple to learn and can be used with students in the elementary grades through college. The maps reflect qualitative characteristics of students' thinking. This is quite different from simple recall.

References

Pollock, M B., & Middleton, K (1989). *Elementary school health instruction.* St. Louis: Times Mirror/Mosby College Publishing.

Shuell, T. J (1990). Phases of meaningful learning. *Review of Educational Research, 60,* 531-547.

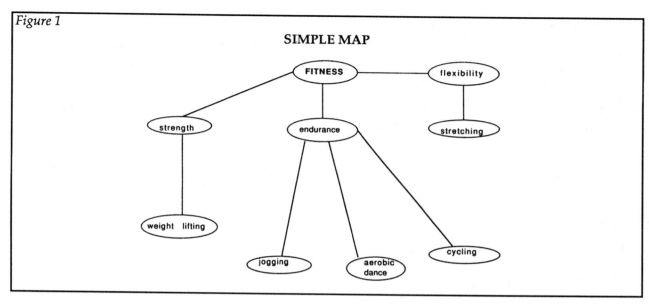

Figure 1

SIMPLE MAP

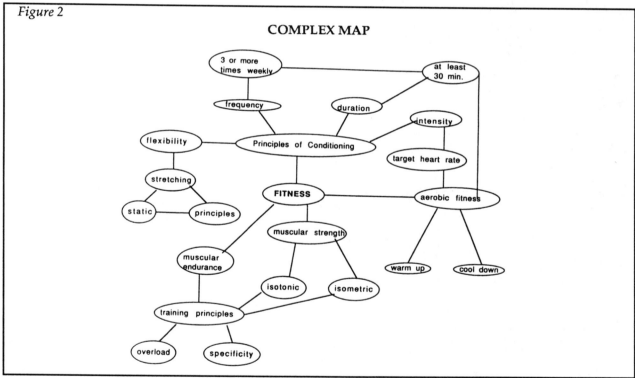

Figure 2

COMPLEX MAP

Purposes of the American Alliance For Health, Physical Education, Recreation and Dance

The American Alliance is an educational organization, structured for the purposes of supporting, encouraging, and providing assistance to member groups and their personnel throughout the nation as they seek to initiate, develop, and conduct programs in health, leisure, and movement-related activities for the enrichment of human life.

Alliance objectives include:

1. Professional growth and development—to support, encourage, and provide guidance in the development and conduct of programs in health, leisure, and movement-related activities which are based on the needs, interests, and inherent capacities of the individual in today's society.

2. Communication—to facilitate public and professional understanding and appreciation of the importance and value of health, leisure, and movement-related activities as they contribute toward human well-being.

3. Research—to encourage and facilitate research which will enrich the depth and scope of health, leisure, and movement-related activities; and to disseminate the findings to the profession and other interested and concerned publics.

4. Standards and guidelines—to further the continuous development and evaluation of standards within the profession for personnel and programs in health, leisure, and movement-related activities.

5. Public affairs—to coordinate and administer a planned program of professional, public, and governmental relations that will improve education in areas of health, leisure, and movement-related activities.

6. To conduct such other activities as shall be approved by the Board of Governors and the Alliance Assembly, provided that the Alliance shall not engage in any activity which would be inconsistent with the status of an educational and charitable organization as defined in Section 501(c)(3) of the Internal Revenue Code of 1954 or any successor provision thereto, and none of the said purposes shall at any time be deemed or construed to be purposes other than the public benefit purposes and objectives consistent with such educational and charitable status.

Bylaws, Article III